HIGH-INTENSITY HOME TRAINING

Learn how to plan, persist, and adapt for larger and stronger muscles.

The massive arm of Paul Dillett.

HIGH-INTENSITY HOME TRAINING

BY ELLINGTON DARDEN, PH.D.
WITH SPECIAL PHOTOGRAPHY BY CHRIS LUND

A Perigee Book

Perigee Books
are published by
The Putnam Publishing Group
200 Madison Avenue
New York, NY 10016

Library of Congress
Cataloging-in-Publication Data

Darden, Ellington, Date
High-intensity home training /
   by Ellington Darden :
with special photography by Chris Lund.
      p. cm.
   ISBN 0-399-51840-1 (acid-free paper)
   1. Weight training. 2. Physical fitness.
   3. Exercise.
I. Lund, Chris.   II. Title
GV546. D274 1993 93   15557 CIP
613.7' 13-dc20

Book design by Martin Moskof;
   book design assistant, George Brady;
   typestyling, Ken Clebanoff;
Cover design by Andrew M. Newman

Printed in the United States of America

1 2 3 4 5 6 7 8 9 10

This book is printed on acid-free paper.

∞

Other Books of Interest
by Ellington Darden, Ph.D.

Big
Massive Muscles in 10 Weeks
Super High-Intensity Bodybuilding
The Nautilus Diet
The Athlete's Guide to Sports Medicine
The Nautilus Bodybuilding Book
The Nautilus Advanced Bodybuilding Book
The Six-Week Fat-To-Muscle Makeover
Big Arms in Six Weeks
100 High-Intensity Ways to Improve
   Your Bodybuilding
32 Days to a 32-Inch Waist
Two Weeks to a Tighter Tummy
New High-Intensity Bodybuilding
Bigger Muscles in 42 Days
Soft Steps to a Hard Body
High-Intensity Strength Training
Grow

WARNING!
The high-intensity routines in this book are intended
only for healthy men and women. People with health
problems should not follow these routines without a
physician's approval. Before beginning any exercise
or dietary program, always consult with your doctor.

PHOTO CREDITS:
Front cover photo of Porter Cottrell and Kevin Levrone
and back cover photo of Flex Wheeler by Chris Lund.
All interior photos by Chris Lund except as noted:
Ellington Darden: 53 / Inge Cook: 57,74,75 / Ken
Hutchins: 143.

A lean midsection requires intelligent eating and
exercising.

CONTENTS

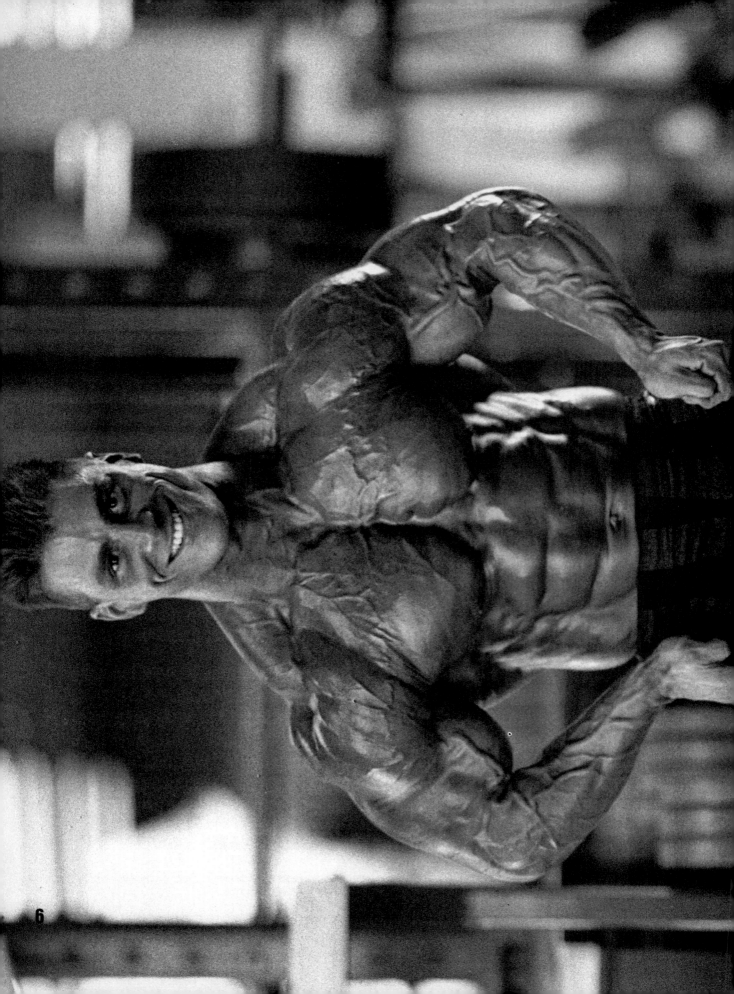

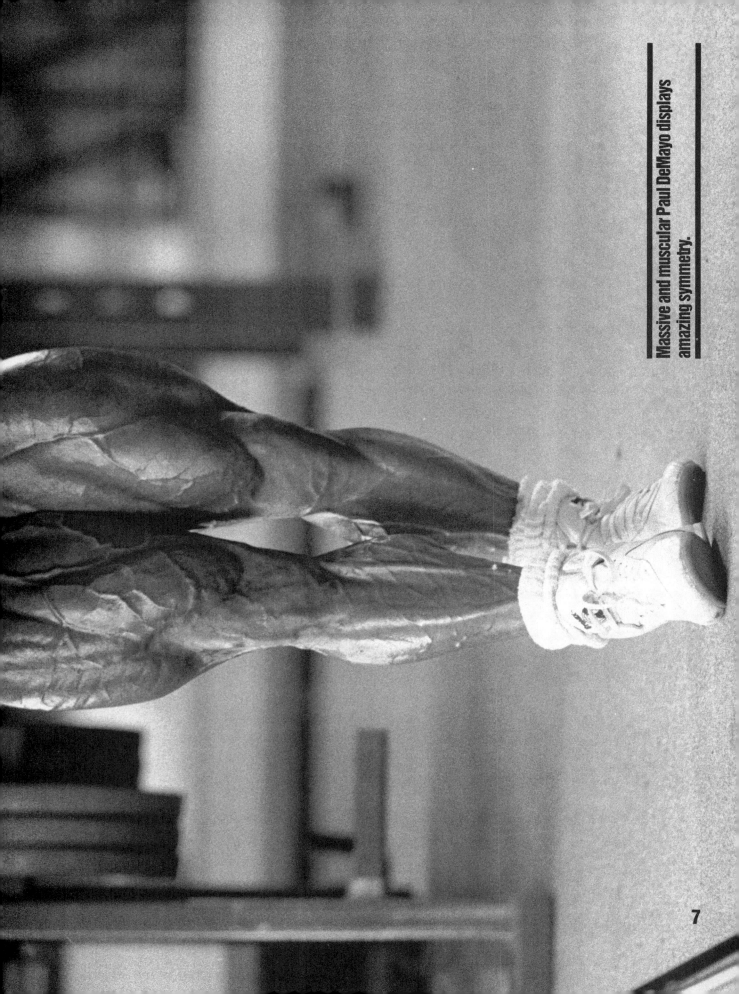

Massive and muscular Paul DeMayo displays amazing symmetry.

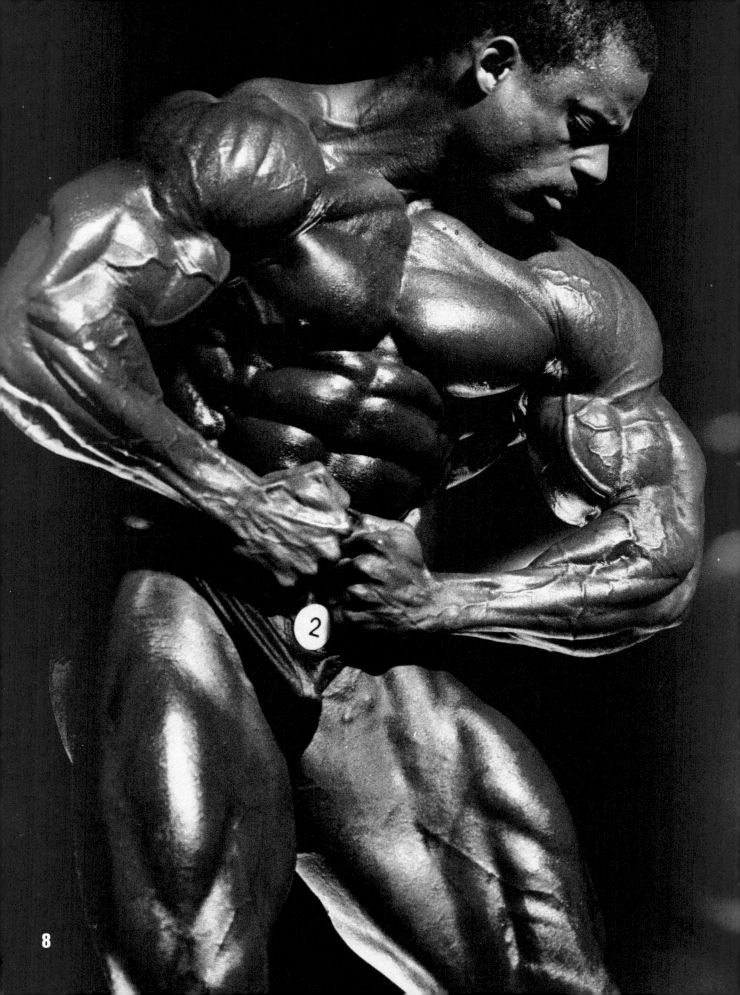

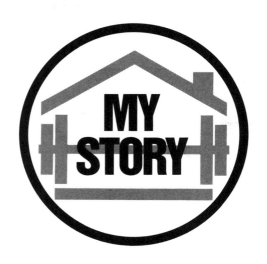

INTRODUCTION

It was June of 1959, and I was fifteen years old. I was five feet nine inches tall and weighed 130 pounds. While I wasn't exactly a skinny beanpole, my body definitely could have improved with some added mass.

After looking through several muscle magazines, I figured lifting weights would add size to my frame. As a result, I purchased a 110-pound combination barbell-dumbbell set for $29.95 at the local sporting goods store.

By coincidence, two of my neighborhood buddies also had bought weights and decided to begin a training program. Soon we consolidated our equipment in one side of my family's two-car garage. We were all rank beginners, so we resorted to the literature that was included with the barbell sets. I can still remember those illustrations of John Grimek, George Jowett, and Sigmund Klein. The photos must have been taken at least

Vince Taylor contracts his rock-hard body.

twenty years earlier, because they all wore those old-time strongman sandals.

GARAGE TRAINING

For six weeks, we performed one set of approximately twelve basic exercises, such as the squat, pullover, calf raise, overhead press, and curl. We trained three times per week.

For the next six weeks, we progressed to two sets and added a few more exercises. Each of our workouts took almost an hour to complete.

Finally, the third six-week course involved doing three sets of each exercise. The new exercises included some weightlifting movements, such as the clean-and-jerk, snatch, and one-armed bent press.

The weightlifting movements gave us all problems. Once, when I was trying to perform a one-armed lift with seventy-five pounds, I lost control of the barbell and it smashed one of my mom's best flowerpots. Within seconds she was in the garage going through a tirade of why we should be more careful with our pot-breaking barbells.

We listened attentively, but we were obsessed with seeing how much we could lift over our heads with one arm. Even today, I still have a catch in my shoulder as a result of my early one-armed lifting.

Nevertheless, all three of us continued to train in my garage for the duration of the summer of 1959.

GETTING ATTENTION

Our progress was steady. Each of us put on from five to ten pounds of muscle, and increased strength in most of the exercises by 50 percent.

When school resumed in the fall, we all

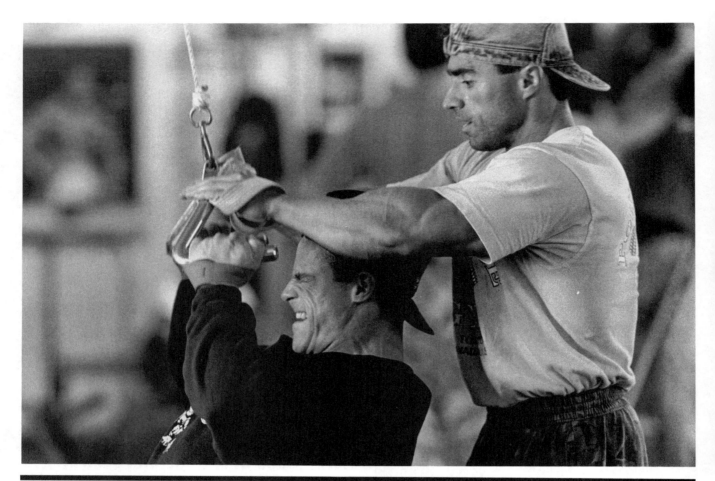

You'll get more efficient results by teaming up with an enthusiastic training partner.

wore tapered black T-shirts that we had ordered from California. Thank goodness a few students noticed our newly built muscles. That little attention certainly helped our motivation.

Unfortunately, my two buddies soon lost interest in training. This actually spurred me on to stick with the weights. I had experienced the results, and I wasn't about to quit.

METALWORKING CLASSES

The other thing that was a significant help was an elective class I took in high school that fall. I had intended to take Woodworking I during my freshman year. To my disappointment, all the classes were full and I was assigned instead to Metalworking I.

Metalworking turned out to be one of my favorite classes, and over the next two years I learned how to weld, build, and cast most of my home-gym equipment. When I graduated from high school in the spring of 1962, I had one of the best home gyms in the state of Texas. Best of all, my body weight had grown from 130 to 205, an improvement of seventy-five pounds. While all of the increase wasn't solid tissue, at least 80 percent of the mass was muscle.

COLLEGE DAYS

Over the next five years, I continued my training in the college town of Waco, Texas. There I exercised in the Baylor University weight room, the local YMCA, and a commercial fitness center. I was introduced to a wider variety of benches and I enjoyed the use of Olympic bars and ready-assembled barbells and dumbbells. But with a little ingenuity, I could have duplicated almost any of these tools in my home gym.

The same training environment was prevalent when I enrolled in graduate school at Florida State University in 1968. For five years, while finishing a Ph.D. in exercise science, I trained on equipment similar to what I had been accustomed to in Texas. It was only during the last year in Tallahassee that equipment took a major turn for the better.

What changed the weight-training equipment business?

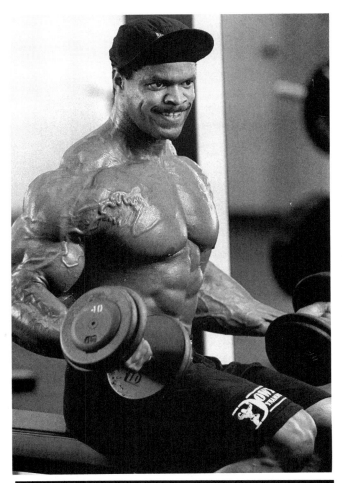

Dumbbells are a versatile muscle-building tool.

ARTHUR JONES

A man named Arthur Jones brought about the change. Jones, a world traveler who was interested in bodybuilding, began to write high-intensity training articles for Iron Man magazine. His articles challenged bodybuilders to train harder but briefer. To do so in the most productive manner, a trainee had to utilize rotary, direct, and variable resistance. Such resistance could be found only in Nautilus machines, which Jones had begun to manufacture.

I worked with Arthur Jones for twenty years, and I can testify to the effectiveness of his philosophy and machines. What I learned and experienced with Nautilus, in fact, has direct application with all home equipment.

Most trainees have some of their best rates of growth during their beginning months of exercising. Why? Because they are practicing an intense program of basic movements. Because they are doing total body workouts only three times per week. Because they are not overtraining.

It is usually when a trainee starts doing multiple sets, split and double-split routines, and maximum attempts that his progress slows, or perhaps he becomes injured. Either way, his enthusiasm drops.

Over ten years of research with Nautilus equipment proved to me that harder, briefer exercise is the key to muscular growth. The same harder, briefer exercise applies to home equipment.

LEARN AND GROW

I wish I had understood during my first years of training what I understand now. I would have saved myself a lot of time, money, frustration, and injuries. And I'd have got-

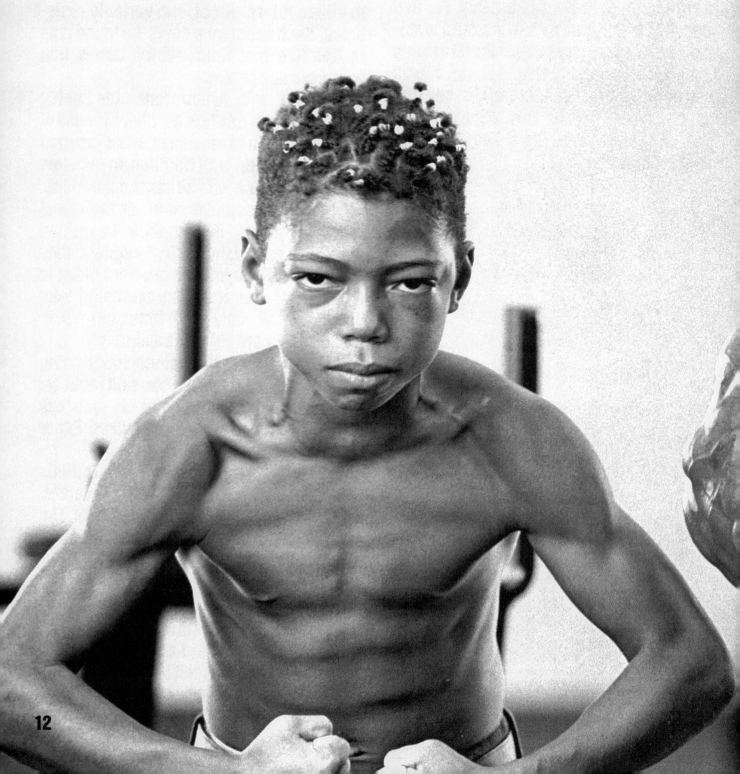

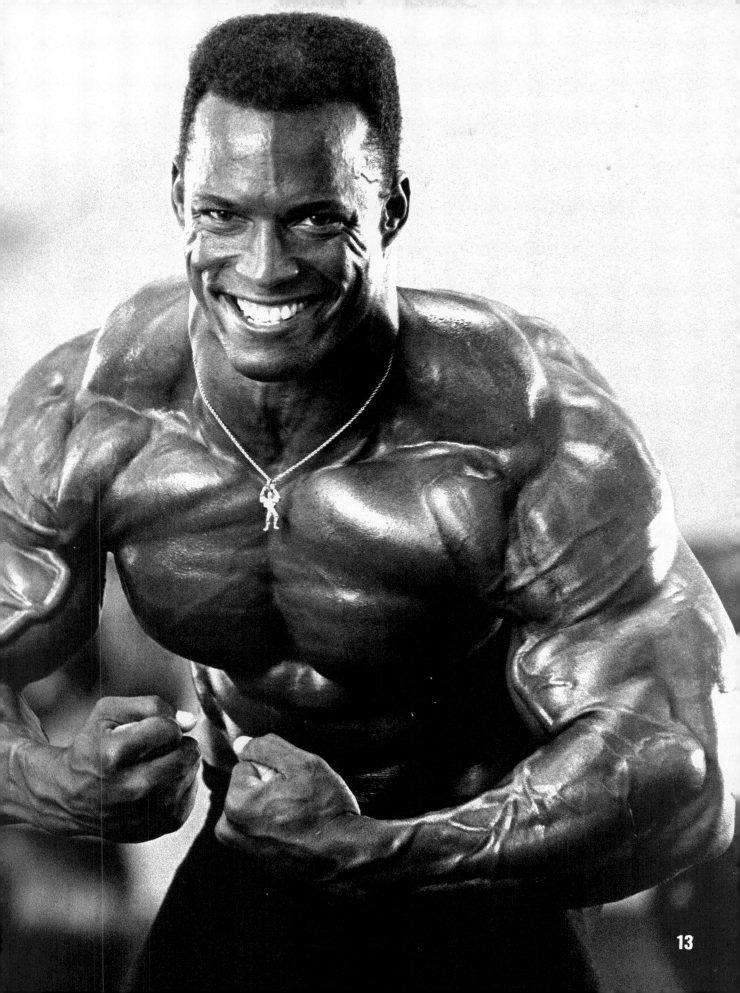

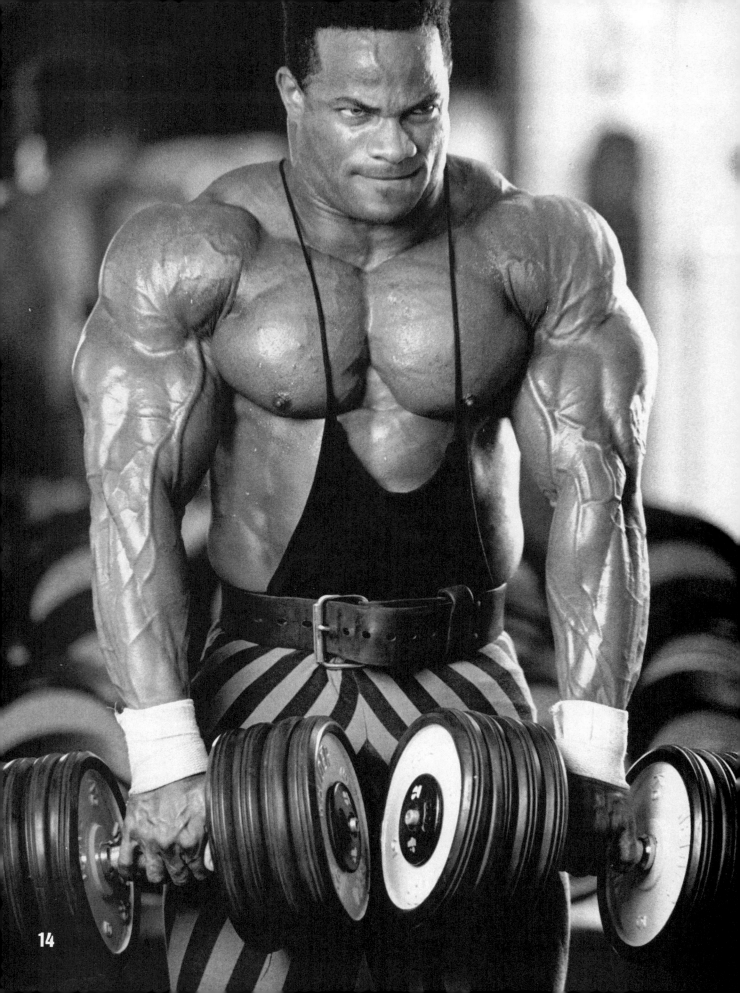

ten several times the muscle-building results in a much shorter period.

In fact, that last statement is the primary purpose of this manual. With the correct application of the high-intensity guidelines, your muscles will get bigger and stronger faster than they will through any other method of exercising with home equipment.

EQUIPMENT NEEDS

The basic home equipment that you'll need for this course is as follows:

- **An adjustable barbell and two dumbbells.** A 110-pound combination barbell-dumbbell set should work fine for a while. In time, however, you will require four additional twenty-five-pound plates.

- **Bench.** A sturdy, adjustable bench with uprights is an important purchase.

- **Squat racks.** The kind that bolt onto the wall are less expensive than freestanding squat stands. Either style, however, will work well.

- **Calf-raise block.** A piece of sturdy wood measuring 18 inches by 4 inches nailed to the top of two 18-inch, 1-inch, by 8-inch boards placed across either end of the 4-by-4 is essential for a variety of calf raises.

- **Chinning bar.** A high horizontal bar in the corner of a room or in a doorway makes a great tool for doing chin-ups.

- **Parallel bars.** Sturdy parallel bars that attach to the wall are an excellent investment.

- **Optional equipment.** Other equipment you may already have access to or want to add

are a lat machine, sit-up board, leg curl machine, and leg extension machine. In addition, it's nice to have handy a big wall clock with a sweeping second hand and a full-length mirror. The clock allows you to time your repetitions, sets, and workouts. The mirror helps you improve your form in certain exercises and gives you visual feedback on your muscle-building progress.

If you're like most home-gym trainees, you'll always be on the lookout for a new piece of equipment. Great! Just remember to buy quality products. Don't be fooled by highly advertised gym gimmicks that promise big muscles with little effort.

THE VERSATILE BARBELL

You don't need gimmicks or fancy machines to get outstanding results. The principles of high-intensity training, which can be performed with any tool, are more important than the implement.

In these days of modern fitness centers with dozens of muscle-building machines, don't laugh at the barbell in the home gym. For the cost, you can't beat the barbell's effectiveness and versatility. Remember, how you lift the weight is more important than the type of weights you use.

The rest of this book will provide you with all the essentials for building massive muscles—in the convenience of your own home.

Get ready to get bigger and stronger NOW!

Alq Gurley does the shoulder shrug with dumbbells in excellent form by keeping his arms straight.

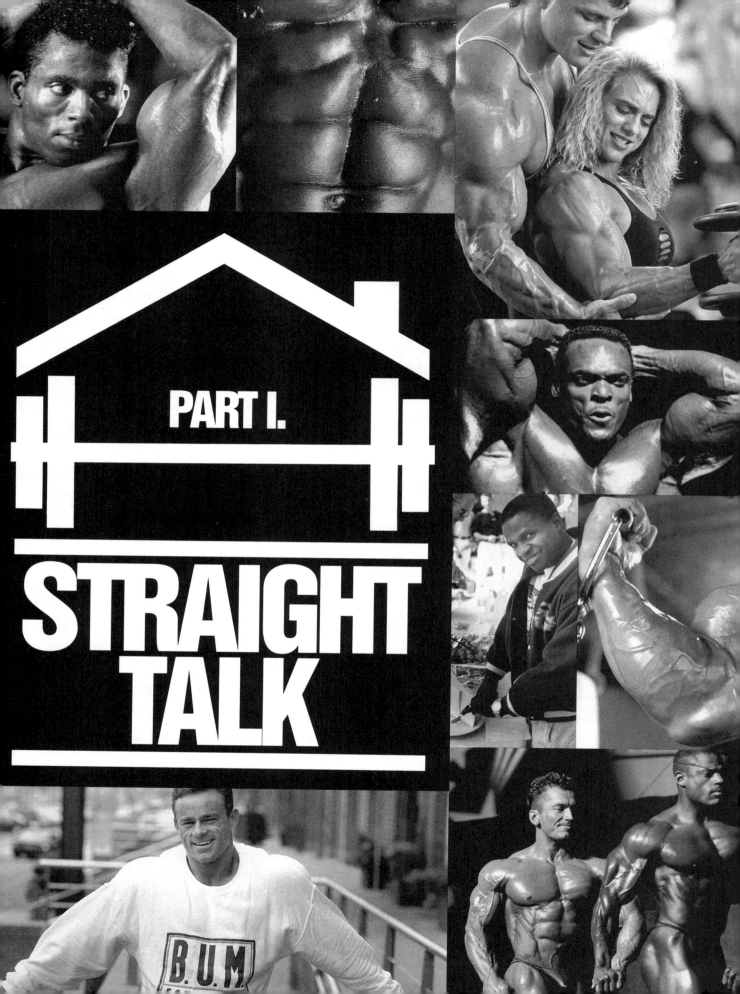

PART I.

STRAIGHT TALK

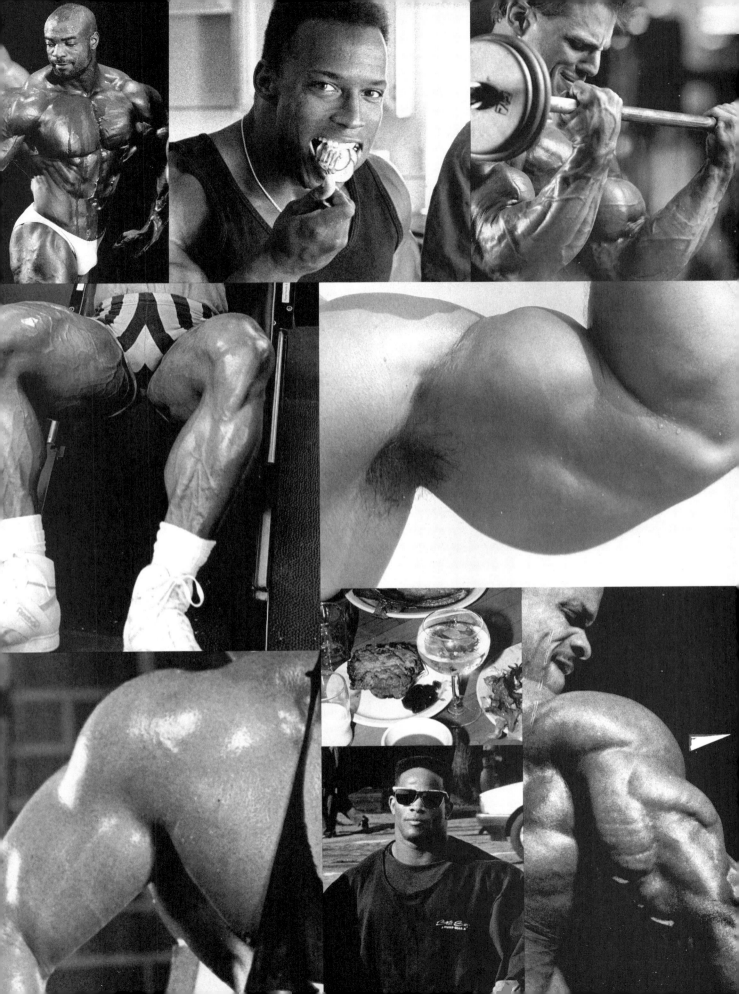

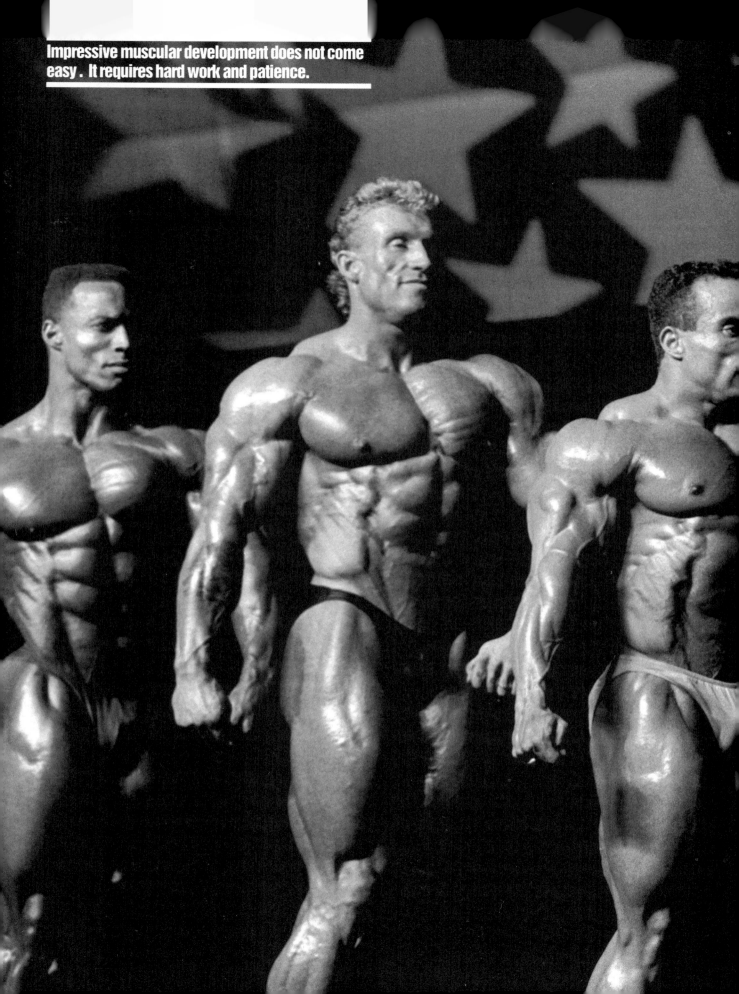

Impressive muscular development does not come easy. It requires hard work and patience.

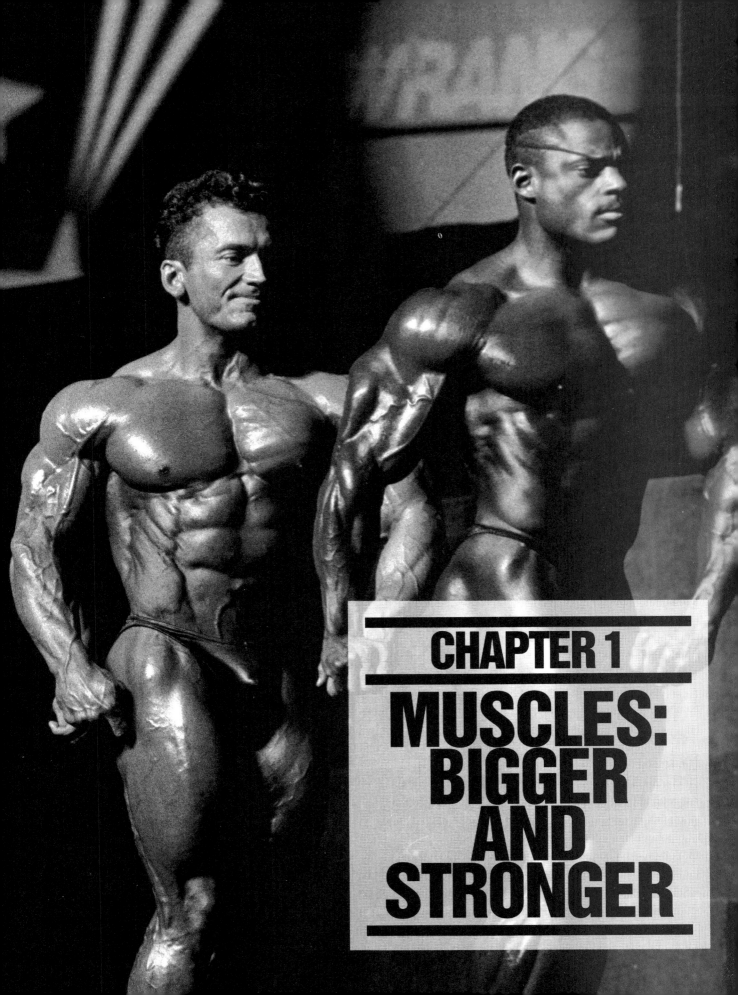

CHAPTER 1
MUSCLES: BIGGER AND STRONGER

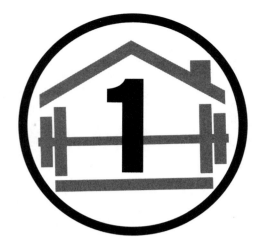

You would like to have:

- ❑ Bigger arms
- ❑ A more massive chest
- ❑ Broader shoulders
- ❑ A V-shaped back
- ❑ Stronger legs

Yes, you can achieve any or all of these goals. You can accomplish these changes much faster if you first understand the structure and function of your body.

Let's roll up our sleeves and get started.

CELLS OF THE HUMAN BODY

Your body is composed of billions of cells: muscle, nerve, blood, fat, and bone. The different kinds of cells perform specific functions. For example, muscle cells can contract and lengthen; they move your body. Blood cells transport oxygen and wastes. Fat cells store energy.

The cell is to your body what a grain of sand is to a sand castle. The cell is your body's smallest unit of structure. Most cells are too small to be seen without a microscope. For instance, as many as 3,000 blood cells lined up side by side measure one inch.

A collection of cells of one type is known as a tissue. Tissues may be combined in one unit or organ where they work together for a specific purpose. The highest level of organ grouping is called a body system. In a body system, organs work together to carry on important bodily functions. All activities dealing with food, for instance, are the responsibility of your digestive system (this is detailed in Chapter 3). For now, however, let's take a brief look at your skeletal and muscular systems.

THE SKELETAL SYSTEM

Your body's skeleton is surrounded by muscles, fat, and skin. The skeleton itself is made up of more than 200 bones that support tissues and protect organs such as the heart and lungs.

Your bones and muscles make it possible for you to move. Tough bands of tissue, called ligaments, connect your bones at the joints. An example of a joint that permits movement in many directions is the ball-and-socket joint of the hip. The ball-shaped end of your thighbone rolls in the socket-type hipbone. Your leg can swing in many different directions because of the construction of this joint.

A joint that permits movement in one direction only is called a hinge joint. There are hinge joints in your knees, elbows, and fingers.

The movement of bone against bone would be difficult if it were not for tissues that almost eliminate friction. Each bone in a joint is coated with a layer of cartilage, which is an elasticlike tissue that has a very smooth surface.

When your forearms and hands move toward your shoulders the biceps muscles of your upper arms contract.

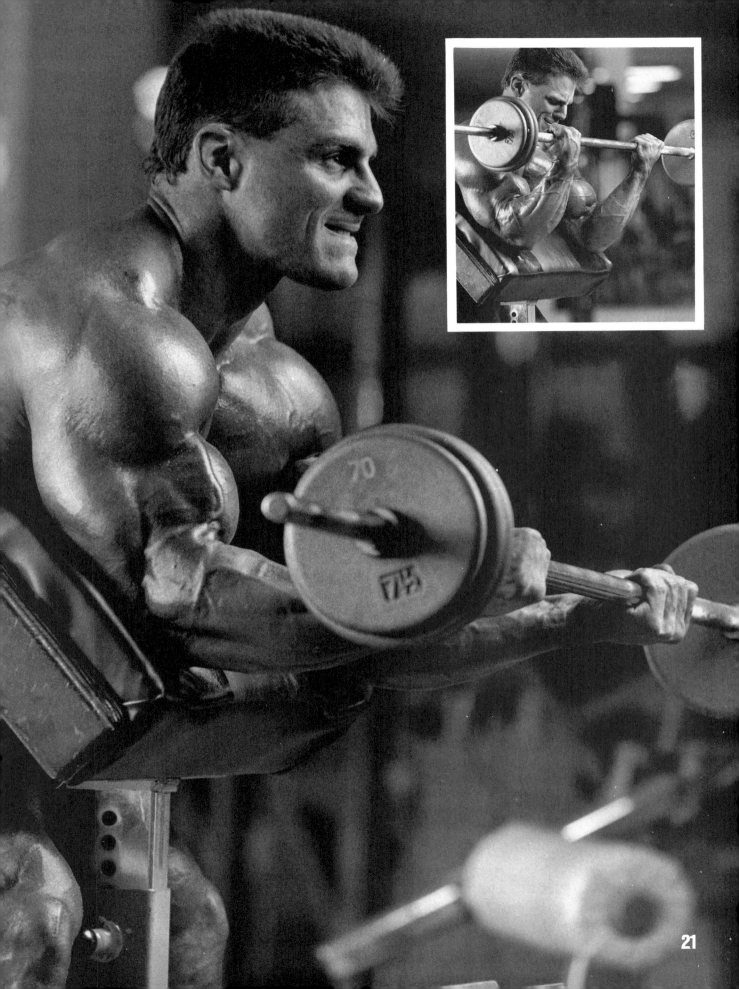

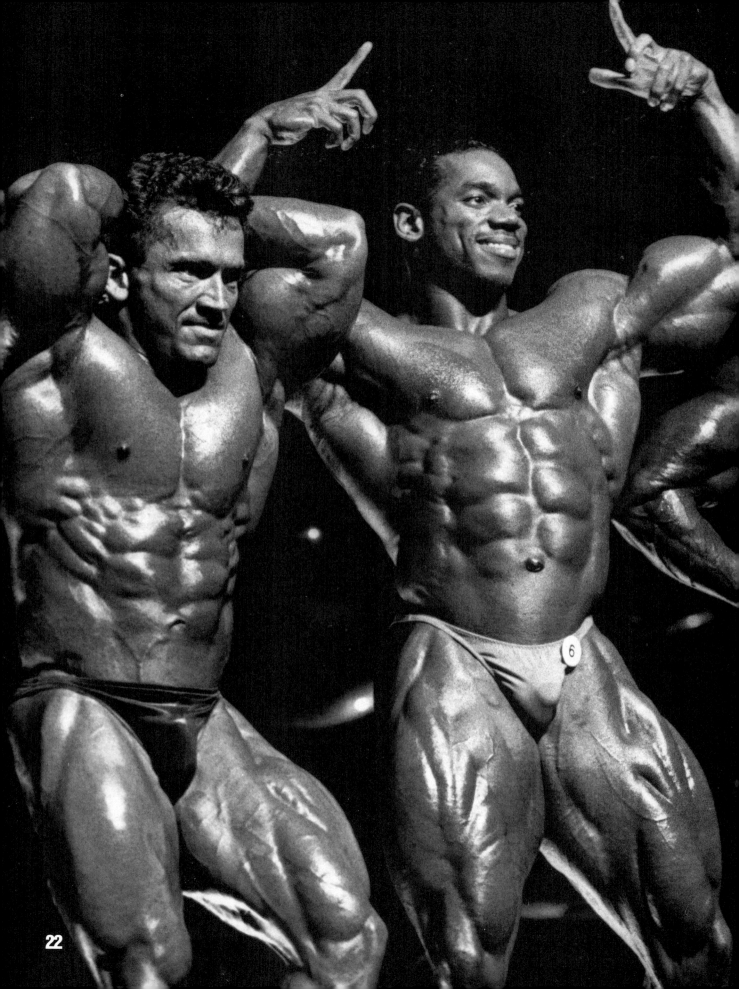

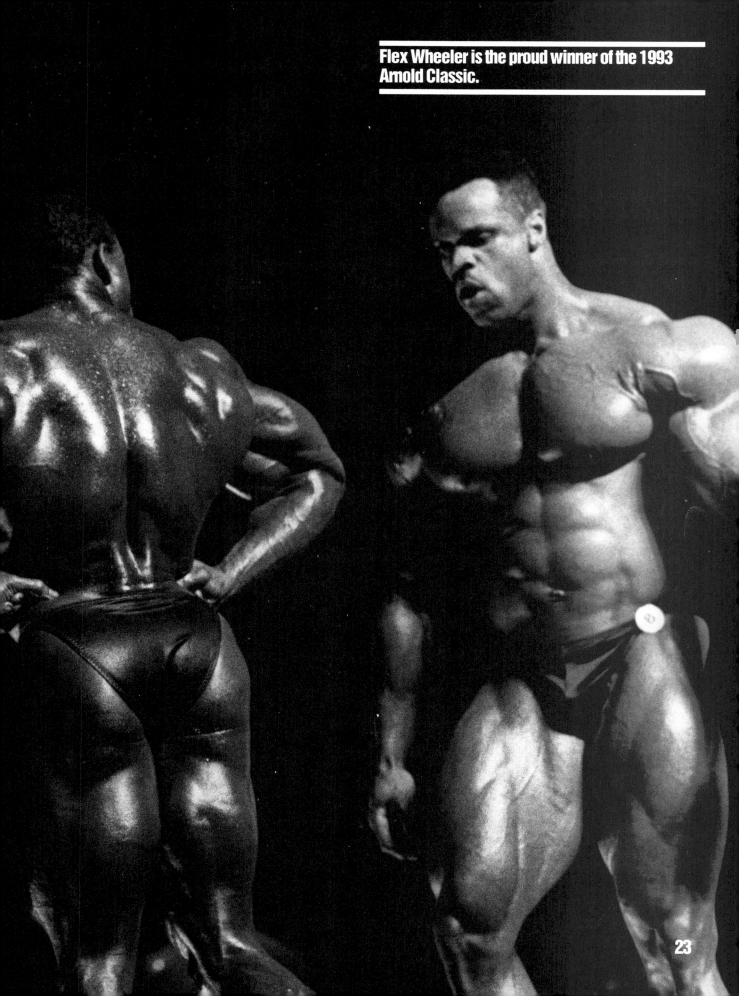

Flex Wheeler is the proud winner of the 1993 Arnold Classic.

During the years of growth, the ends of the long bones of your body are fastened to the shafts, mainly by a wide cartilage band known as the growth plate (epiphysis). Bone cells gradually develop from the shaft. They start displacing the cartilage cells by turning into hard, new bone cells. The cartilage cells are then forced to move toward the ends of the long bones. As the cartilage moves outward, the long bones grow. By the time you have reached age eighteen to twenty, the growth plates have all turned to bone, or ossified, and you can grow no taller.

"Stay away from weightlifting," say some authorities. "It will stunt your growth." This warning used to keep teenagers away from weights because heavy exercise might damage the growth plates of the long bones.

There is legitimate concern on this issue. However, according to recent recommendations by the American Academy of Pediatrics, the American Orthopaedic Society for Sports Medicine, and the American College of Sports Medicine, teenagers do not have to avoid lifting weights altogether; instead, they should avoid trying to see how much they can lift in a one-time, all-out effort. The organizations above are opposed to young people doing Olympic lifting (clean-and-jerk and snatch) and power lifting (squat, bench press, and deadlift). Instead, they suggest that young people train with submaximum weights. They should select a weight they can perform eight to twelve times.

Weight training performed in this manner is suggested throughout this book. Such training has a very beneficial effect on a youngster's skeletal and muscular systems.

THE MUSCULAR SYSTEM

Muscles exist in three types. The muscles used for voluntary body movements are skeletal muscle. The heart, automatically operated by the nervous system and not under conscious control, is composed of cardiac muscle. A third type, called smooth muscle, automatically serves internal functions. They push food through the stomach and intestines and constrict blood vessels to adjust blood flow.

Most of the muscle tissue in your body is voluntary skeletal muscle. Billions of cells are packed into fiber bundles, which combine to make even larger bundles. At the smallest microscopic level inside your muscle fibers are thick and thin protein strands called myosin and actin. It is at this microscopic level that the actual growth of your muscle occurs. Proper weight training stimulates the formation of more myosin and actin. More myosin and actin lead to more protein filaments, which in turn results in larger muscle fibers. Larger muscle fibers then produce greater muscular size and strength in the involved fiber bundles, such as your biceps, deltoids, and quadriceps.

There are 424 skeletal muscles in your body. They normally account for between one-third and one-half of your body weight, depending on your age, sex, and the amount of fat on your body. Your muscles work together to do many things, such as standing, walking, running, breathing, eating, laughing, and sleeping. Muscles work in harmony with your skeletal system. Neither system could do its job without the other.

MUSCLE-FIBER TYPE

Although over a dozen different classifications of muscle fibers have been discovered within the human body, scientists generally group them into two types. These two types refer to fatigueability, or how slow or how fast a muscle tires.

The first type is called slow-twitch fiber, because it is slow to contract but has the ability to continue working for long periods of time. People who have a high percentage of slow-twitch fiber usually excel as long-distance cyclists, swimmers, and runners.

The second fiber type is called fast-twitch, which is best suited for short-term, powerful contractions. Individuals with a high percentage of fast-twitch fiber perform well as throwers, sprinters, and jumpers.

Individuals vary in the number of slow-twitch and fast-twitch muscle fibers throughout the body. Individuals with a large percentage of fast-twitch fibers have greater potential for increasing muscular size and strength than individuals with a predominance of slow-twitch fibers. Most people seem to have approximately equal numbers of both slow- and fast-twitch muscle fibers throughout their body. A small number, however, have 90 percent or more from one fiber type.

Whatever your ratio, it is determined genetically and cannot be altered. In fact, the only way to be sure of your fiber type is to undergo a series of muscle biopsies where a small sample of muscle is taken from various body parts and analyzed. Muscle biopsies are not practical for most people. A non-surgical way of estimating your fiber type is described in Chapter 14 of my book High-Intensity Strength Training.

You also need to understand that specific training does not change slow-twitch fibers to fast-twitch fibers or vice versa. Remember, your fiber type is inherited.

Furthermore, there are no differences in fiber-type distribution between males and females. There is no such thing as a male or female muscle fiber. A muscle fiber is a muscle fiber, and slow-and fast-twitch fibers are found in both females and males, with the same distribution and fiber performance characteristics.

WHAT'S NEXT?

For your muscles to get bigger and stronger, three things must happen. First, you must stimulate the targeted muscle to grow at the myosin and actin level. Second, you must permit the stimulated muscle to grow with the necessary recovery and rest. Third, adequate nutrients must be available.

The next two chapters will examine recovery and nutrition.

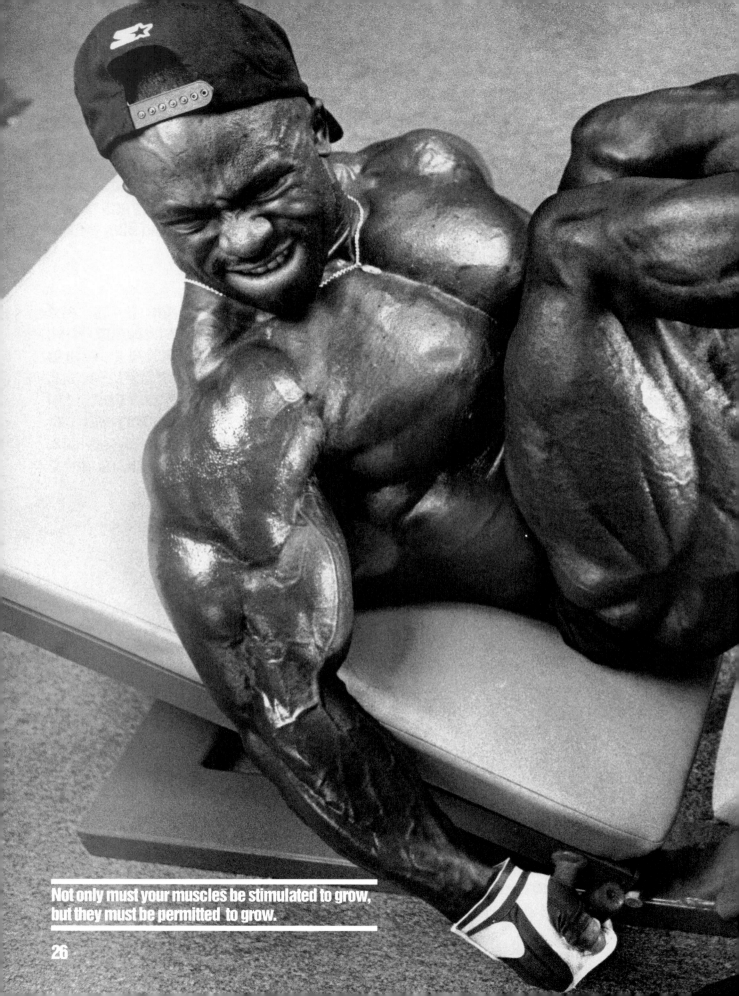

Not only must your muscles be stimulated to grow, but they must be permitted to grow.

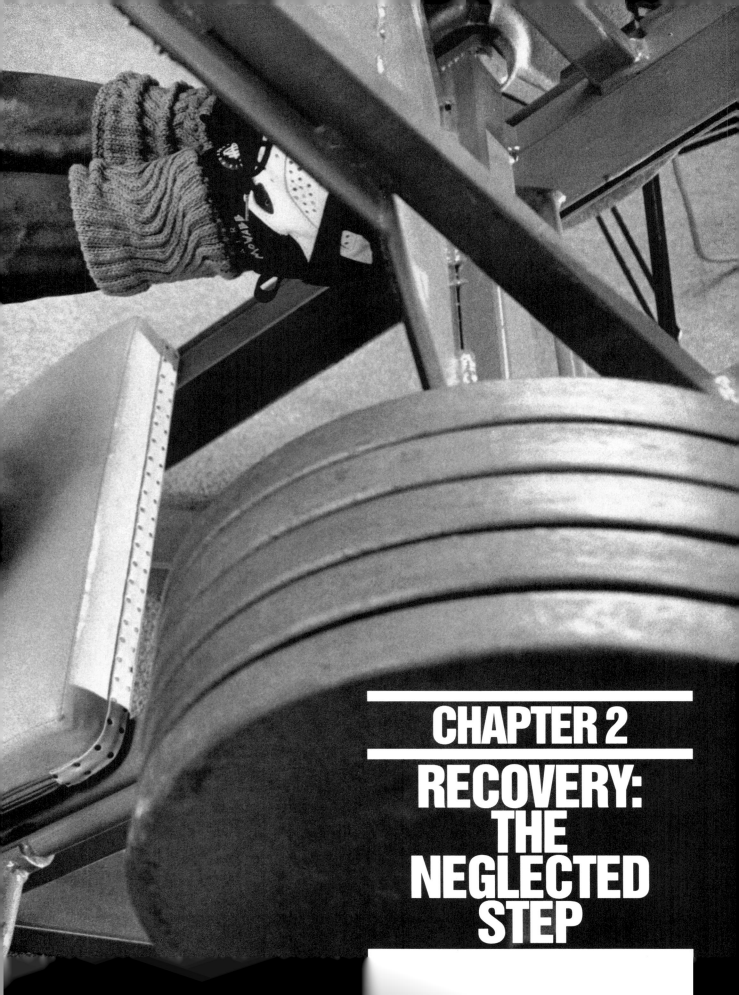

CHAPTER 2
RECOVERY: THE NEGLECTED STEP

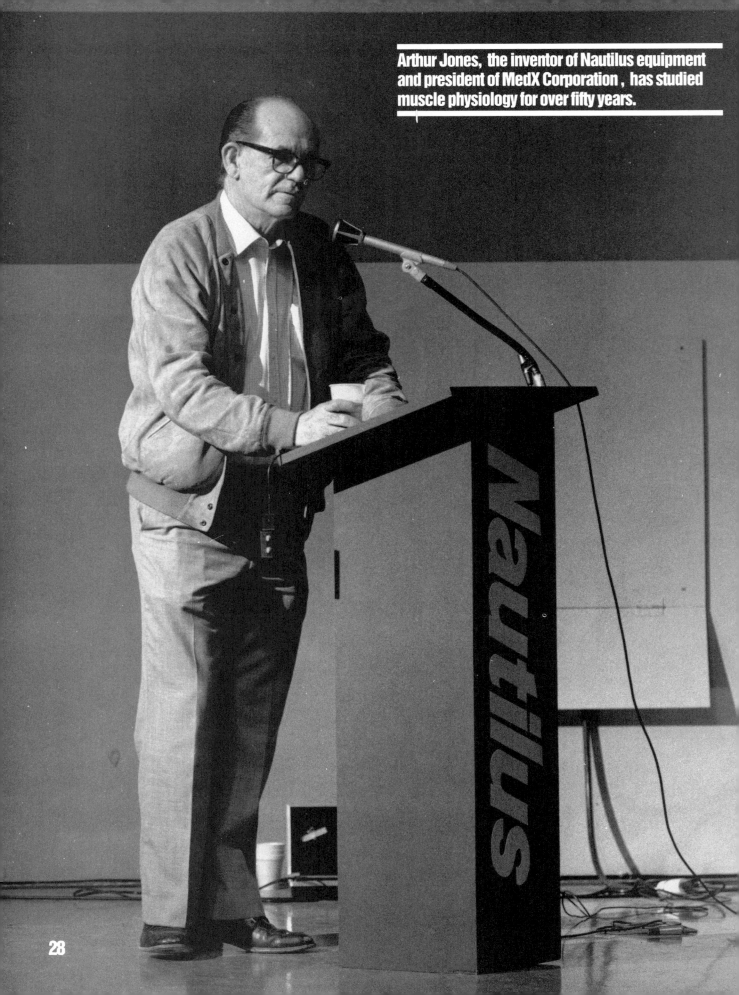

Arthur Jones, the inventor of Nautilus equipment and president of MedX Corporation, has studied muscle physiology for over fifty years.

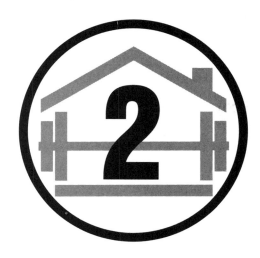

Too many bodybuilders, especially those who've been training for six months or longer, neglect their recovery ability. In other words, they get too little rest and too little sleep between workouts. They often stimulate their muscles to grow, but they seldom get the anticipated results. The reason is directly related to their weakened recovery ability.

RECOVERY ABILITY

Recovery ability is defined as the chemical reactions that are necessary for your body to produce muscular growth. Your body is a complex chemical factory, constantly making hundreds of delicate changes that transform food and oxygen into many elements needed by various parts of the system. But there is a limit to the chemical conversions that your recovery ability can make within a given time. If your requirements exceed that limit, your body will eventually be overwhelmed to the point of collapse.

Thus, an ideal exercise would be infinitely hard and infinitely brief. It would provide maximum growth stimulation while leaving your recovery ability in the best possible shape to meet the requirements for growth.

To illustrate this concept even further, I'd like to rehash a thought-provoking anecdote that I used in Chapter 47 of my book High-Intensity Strength Training. The story involved a challenge that Arthur Jones made to readers of Iron Man magazine during the early 1970s.

THE JONES CHALLENGE

"From only one workout," Arthur Jones promised, "I'll put half an inch of permanent muscle size on your upper arms!" Jones's promise was made to advanced bodybuilders who would do almost anything to add a fraction of an inch to their biceps and triceps.

Furthermore, Jones backed his promise up with a remarkable guarantee: "If you don't put half an inch of solid muscle on your arms, I'll pay your expenses to and from Florida."

As you can imagine, many bodybuilders made the journey to the Nautilus headquarters. I witnessed Jones put dozens of men through his workouts. And crazy as this whole challenge seemed, he actually made good on his promise. I never saw any of these men ask for their expenses to be reimbursed.

What was Jones's secret? How was he able to renew growth so fast?

In a nutshell, the secret was lots of REST and SLEEP!

THE FORMULA

Here's the surefire formula that Arthur Jones devised:

First, Jones would usually meet the arriving bodybuilder at the airport, bus station, or a local restaurant. Almost immediately he'd get out his tape and measure the upper arms. Then, over a large and leisurely meal,

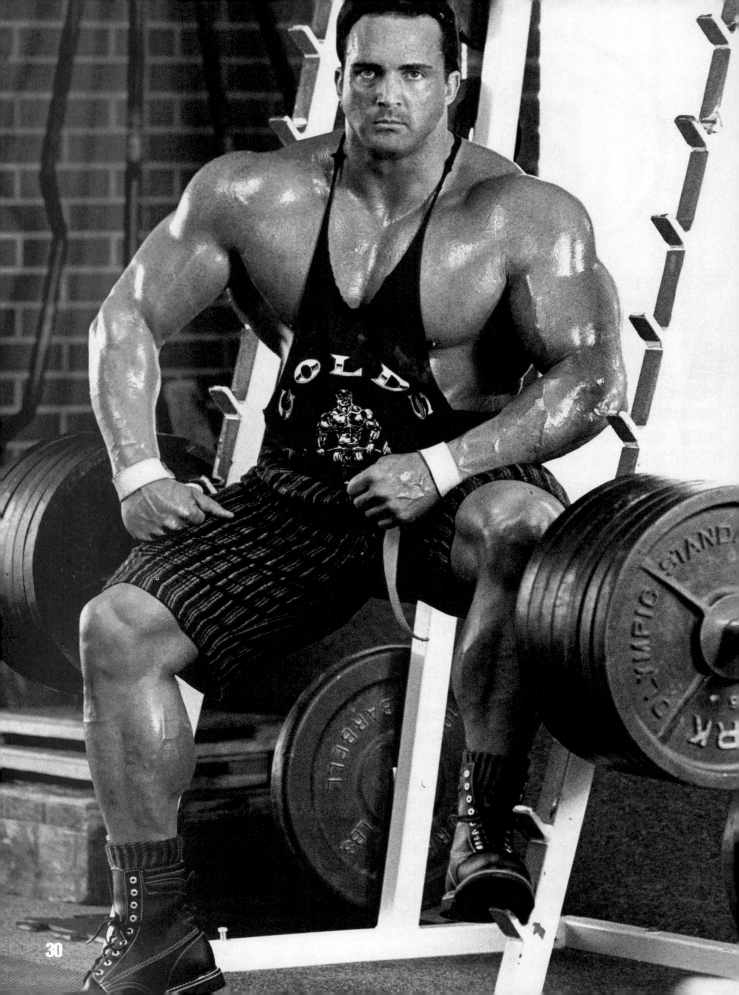

they'd talk training and Jones's harder-but-briefer philosophy.

After several hours of discussion, Jones would check him into a beach-side motel, where he was instructed to spend the next three nights and days sleeping and resting. Invariably, the bodybuilder would ask, "But what about my workout?"

Jones knew from his dinner conversation that the bodybuilder was in a state of over-training—as most were then, and are now—so it would be counterproductive to try to exercise him in that condition. What he desperately needed was rest, relaxation, and sleep—plenty of all three—and no workouts. Yes, he could enjoy the beach, the sun, the surf, and the fresh air. But no, absolutely no, exercise of any kind! And Jones made the guy give him his word on this.

Jones would meet the bodybuilder at the Nautilus training room in DeLand on the afternoon of the fourth day. Talk about being enthusiastic, the guy would usually be almost wild. After training almost every day, often twice a day, for years—the body feels simply great after three days of rest. Before the workout, however, Jones would measure the arms again. With most bodybuilders, their arms would already be 1/4-inch larger. That's right, 1/4-inch bigger from no exercise!

The workout never consisted of more than ten exercises. Usually there were two exercises for the legs, two for the torso, and the rest devoted to the arms. Sometimes Jones skipped working the legs.

Only one set of each was performed, but

Chris Duffy, at a body weight of 280 pounds, is one of the biggest men in bodybuilding.

each exercise was carried to all-out failure. It's impossible to describe the type of failure that Arthur Jones gets out of people, except to say simply: it's extreme! Many of the bodybuilders would throw up after the first three exercises. All of them wanted to. They all took a long rest, flat on their backs or stomachs, after the workout. No one ever asked for a second set of any exercise.

An hour after the workout, and over another meal, Jones was back explaining his new philosophy. It was surprising how much more receptive and inquisitive the body-builder was now. After another hour or two, it was back to the motel for another night's sleep.

Finally, Jones would arrive early the next morning at the motel for climatic measurements. On each one I ever witnessed or heard about, there was at least a 1/2-inch increase on each upper arm. A few gained 5/8 of an inch or more. Only two guys came close to failing. They registered a 7/16-inch increase per arm, but after one more night's sleep, they were up another 1/8 inch.

SALIENT GUIDELINES

I've learned a great deal about strength training from being associated with Arthur Jones for more than twenty years. But nothing I've learned has had more salience than the importance of rest and sleep in building larger and stronger muscles.

I've also read many articles and books on rest and sleep that complement Jones's beliefs. I'm convinced that you'll get better results from your high-intensity strength training if you apply the following guidelines:

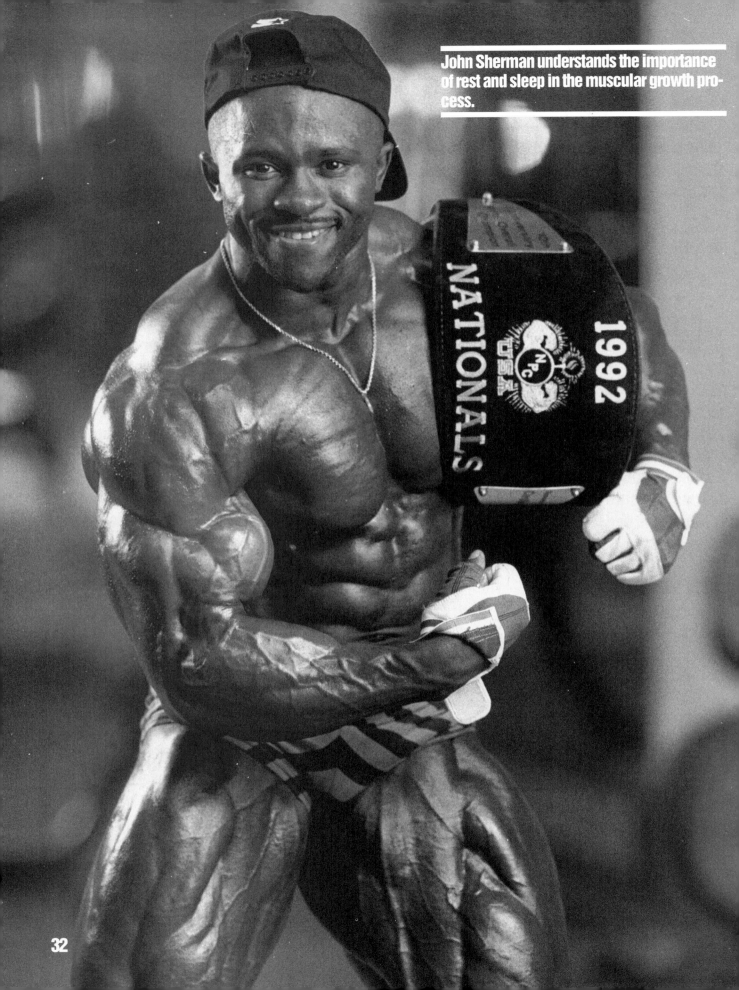

- Get ten hours of sleep each night if you are a teenager.
- Get nine hours of sleep each night if you are an adult.
- Schedule a fifteen-minute nap during the middle of the afternoon, if possible.
- Do not do any type of vigorous activity on your days off.
- Take a ten-day layoff after each period of six months of steady training.

In summary, if you rest and sleep well, your muscles will reward you for it.

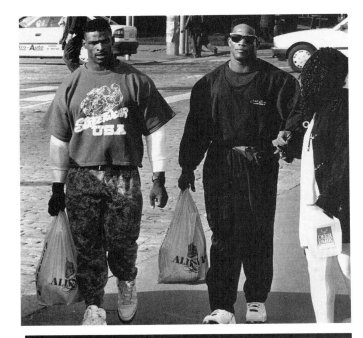

Ronald Coleman and Alq Gurley relax and do a little shopping between contests during the European Grand Prix tour.

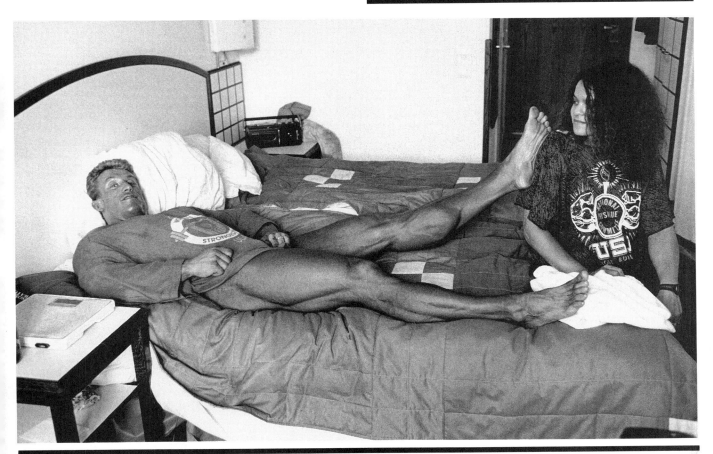

Dorian Yates takes it easy before winning the 1992 Mr. Olympia.

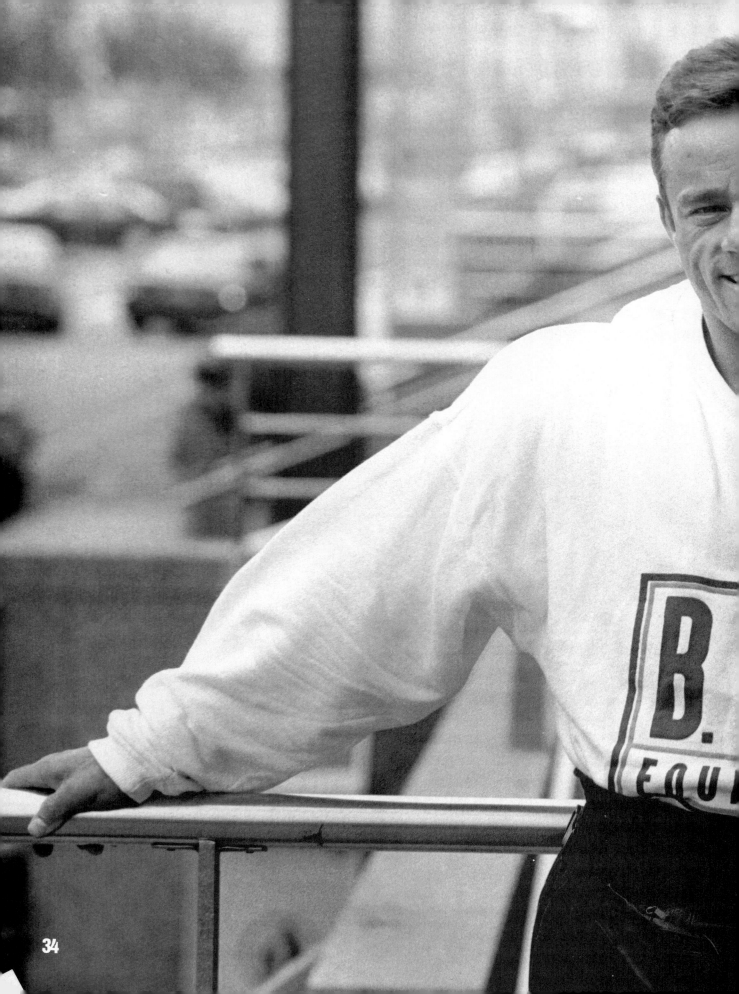

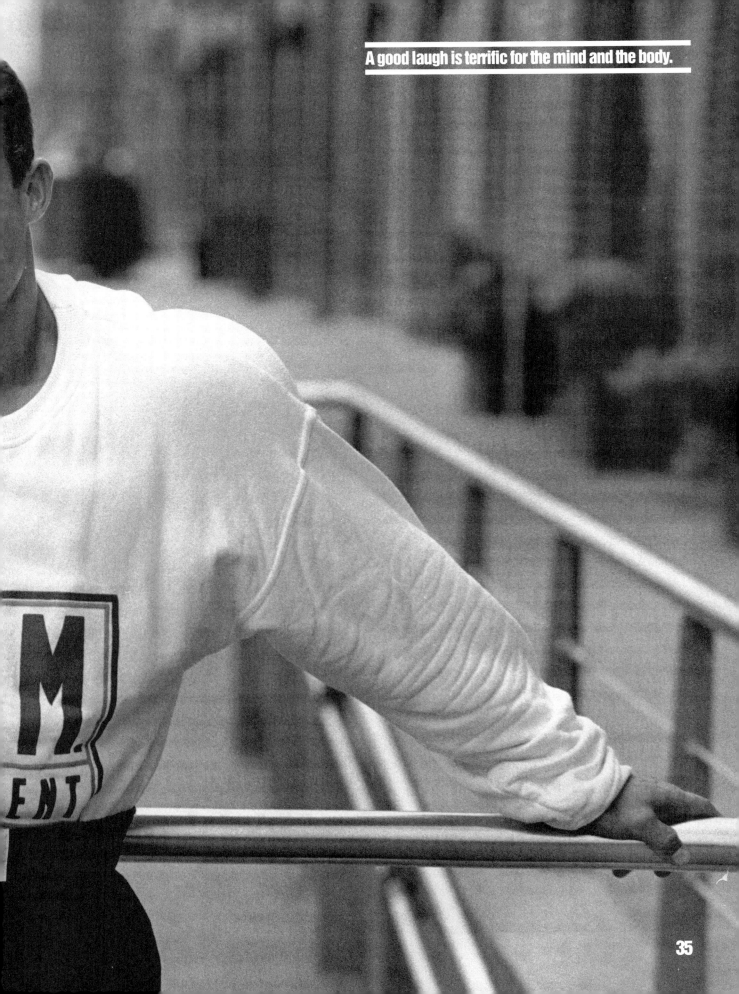

A good laugh is terrific for the mind and the body.

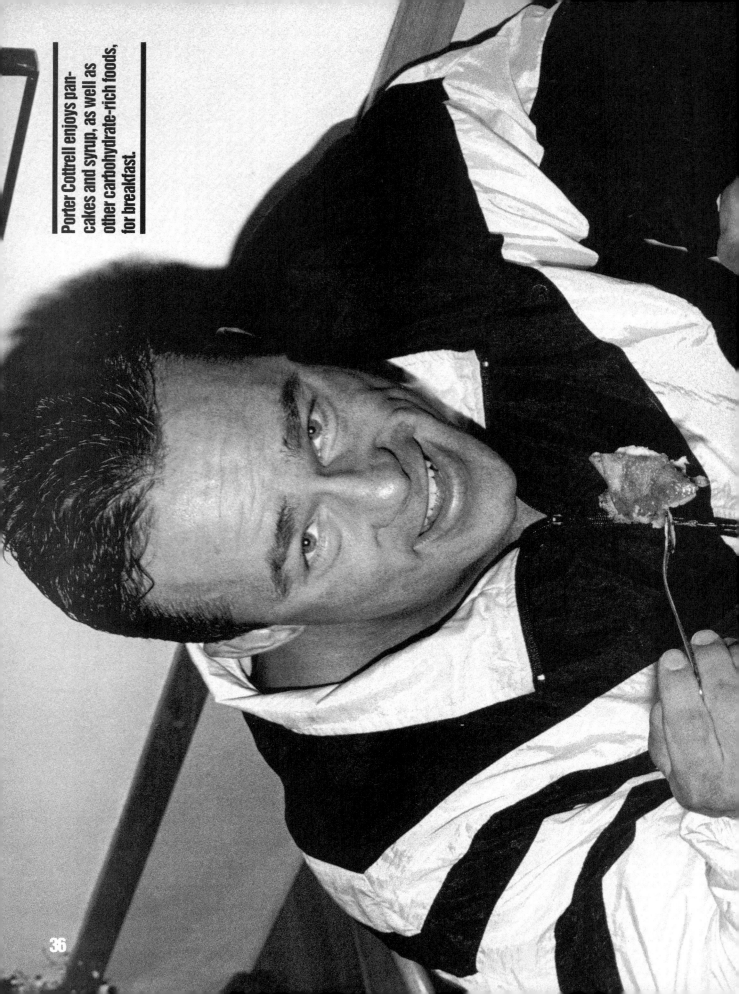

Porter Cottrell enjoys pancakes and syrup, as well as other carbohydrate-rich foods, for breakfast.

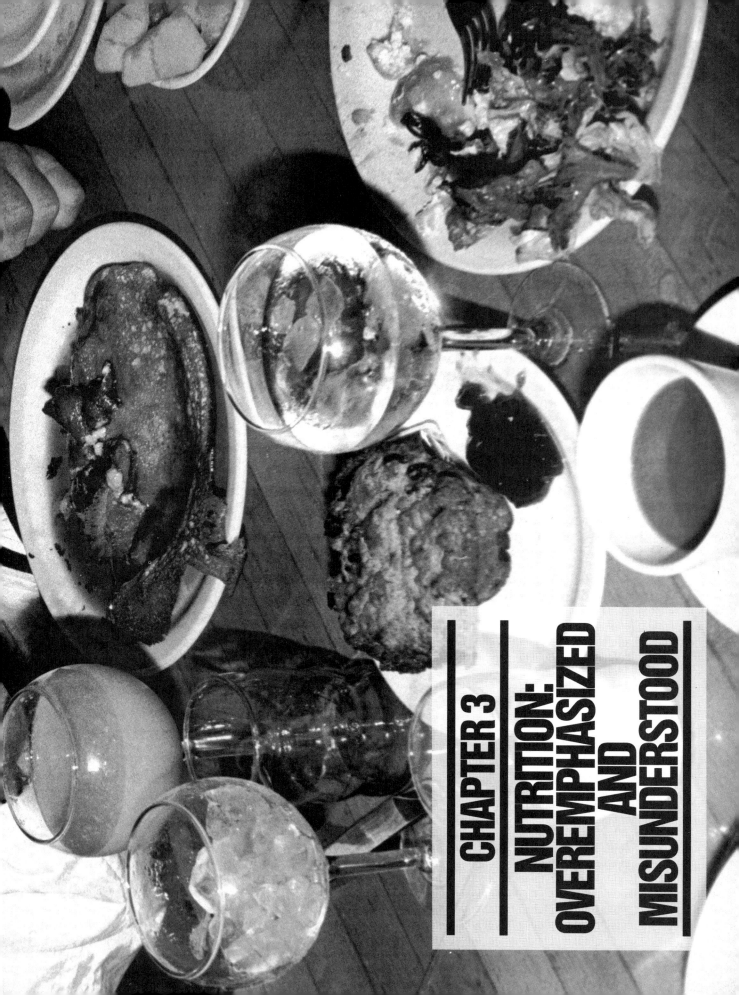

CHAPTER 3
NUTRITION: OVEREMPHASIZED AND MISUNDERSTOOD

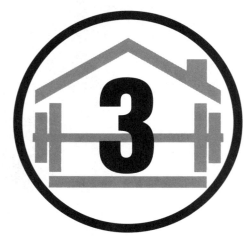

How important is nutrition in the overall process of building larger and stronger muscles?

Research performed twenty years ago at Harvard University by Dr. Alfred Goldberg revealed a startling conclusion. Dr. Goldberg tested groups of laboratory rats for muscular growth under various conditions. In the process he stumbled onto a fundamental biological priority. He found that if stimulated, muscle will grow in spite of tremendous adversity. For example, he noted significant muscular growth could occur on a starvation diet of only water. How was such growth possible? One of the essential traits of animal life is locomotion. Locomotion depends on muscular strength. Survival resources, therefore, are allocated to the working muscles first. This priority allocation, however, is dependent upon muscular growth stimulation. Without stimulation, resources are stored, sloughed off, or put to other uses.

What can you learn from the research with laboratory rats? Simply, if building muscle is your goal, then exercise is much more important than nutrition. Exercise, not food, produces growth stimulation.

SERGIO'S PIZZA AND COKE

In the 1960s and early 1970s, Sergio Oliva

was the most impressive bodybuilder of his day. He won the Mr. Olympia Contest in 1967, 1968, and 1969. He spent part of the summer of 1971 training in Florida under the tutelage of Arthur Jones. Almost every day, Sergio's primary food sources were pizza, which is often condemned for being high in fat calories, and Coca-Cola, which is frequently panned for being loaded with simple sugar.

Sergio reached his peak condition — in fact, his flexed upper arm actually measured bigger than his head — by training extremely hard and consuming so-called junk food. Amazing, to say the least, but true!

The Harvard research and the Sergio example are not meant to imply that food and nutrition are not important. Stop eating for several days and you see how important they are. In my opinion, however, they are certainly overemphasized — especially in bodybuilding magazines. The muscle magazines are crammed full of advertisements for food supplements, most of which are manufactured by the publisher of the magazine. To build massive muscles, your body does not require expensive supplements or exotic foods. Primarily, it requires calories and water. Secondarily, it needs relatively moderate amounts of carbohydrates, proteins, fats, vitamins, and minerals.

A more important question to ask than "What do I need to eat for optimum bodybuilding?" is "What do I need to eat for optimum health and longevity?"

Proper nutrition is the cornerstone of good health. With a few exceptions, what is required for good health is also what is required for muscle building.

Let's explore the latest on healthy eating.

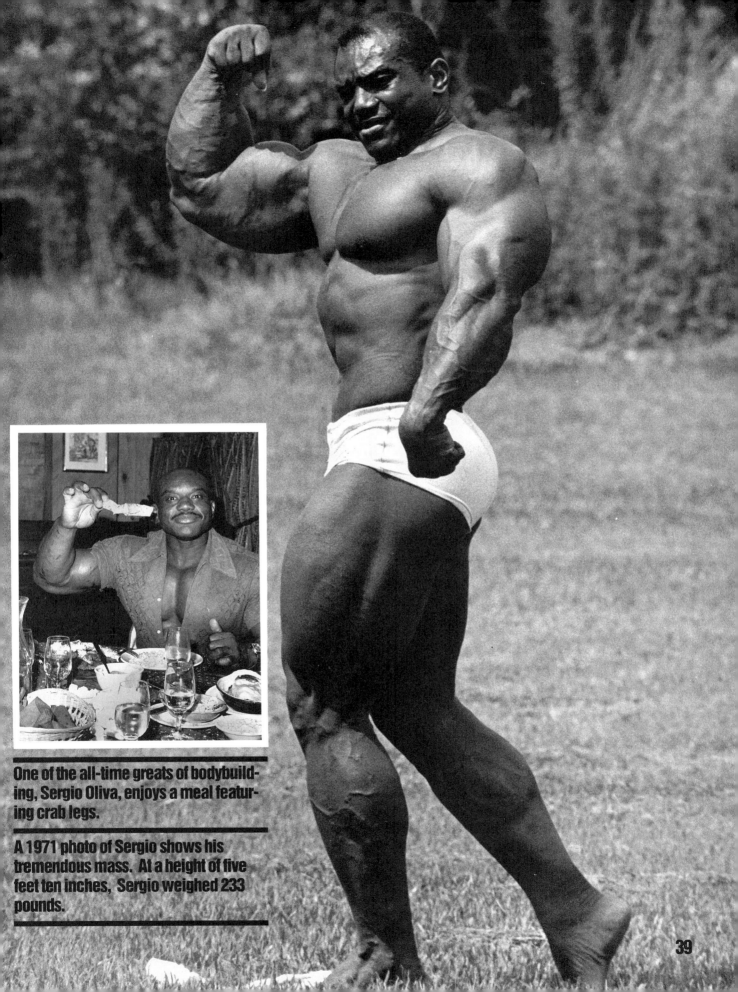

One of the all-time greats of bodybuilding, Sergio Oliva, enjoys a meal featuring crab legs.

A 1971 photo of Sergio shows his tremendous mass. At a height of five feet ten inches, Sergio weighed 233 pounds.

STEPS TO HEALTHY EATING

Over the last several years, Americans have been bombarded with a wide array of nutrition advice. You are no doubt aware that certain dietary changes seem to lower the risk of heart disease and cancer. Yet with all the advice available, it isn't always clear which guidelines are most important and how to apply them on a daily basis.

Study the following steps and incorporate them into your eating plan:

- Keep your total fat intake at or below 30 percent of your daily calories. Limit your intake of fat by selecting lean meats, poultry without skin, fish, and low-fat dairy products. In addition, cut back on vegetable oils and butter—or foods made with these—as well as on mayonnaise, salad dressings, and fried foods.

- Limit your intake of saturated fat to less than 10 percent of your fat calories. A diet high in saturated fat contributes to high blood-cholesterol levels. The richest sources of saturated fat are animal products and tropical vegetable oils, such as coconut or palm oil.

- Decrease your cholesterol intake to 300 milligrams or less per day. Cholesterol is found only in animal products, such as meats, poultry, dairy products, and egg yolks.

- Consume a diet high in complex carbohydrates. Carbohydrates should contribute at least 55 percent of your total daily calories. To help meet this requirement, eat five or more servings of a combination of vegetables and fruits, and six or more servings of whole grains or legumes daily. This will help you obtain the 20 to 30 grams of dietary fiber you need each day, as well as provide important vitamins and minerals.

- Maintain a moderate protein intake. Protein should make up about 12 percent of your total daily calories. Choose low-fat sources of protein.

- Eat a variety of foods. Don't try to fill your nutrient requirements by consuming the same foods every day. Experiment with new and different foods—and read the labels carefully.

- Avoid too much sugar. Many foods that are high in sugar are also high in fat. Sugar also contributes to tooth decay.

- Lower your sodium intake to 2,400 milligrams per day. This is equal to the amount of sodium in a little more than a teaspoon of salt. Cut back on your use of salt in cooking. Avoid salty foods and check food labels for the inclusion of ingredients containing sodium.

- Emphasize an adequate calcium intake. Calcium is essential for strong bones and teeth. Get your calcium from low-fat sources, such as skim milk and low-fat yogurt.

- Get your vitamins and minerals from foods. If you take a vitamin-mineral supplement, make sure it contains no more than the Recommended Dietary Allowance (RDA) for any one nutrient.

- Don't drink alcohol. Excess alcohol consumption can lead to a variety of health problems. And alcoholic beverages can add many calories to your diet without supplying other nutrients.

Applying the tips to healthy eating is easier than you think. Here are some healthy meal recommendations.

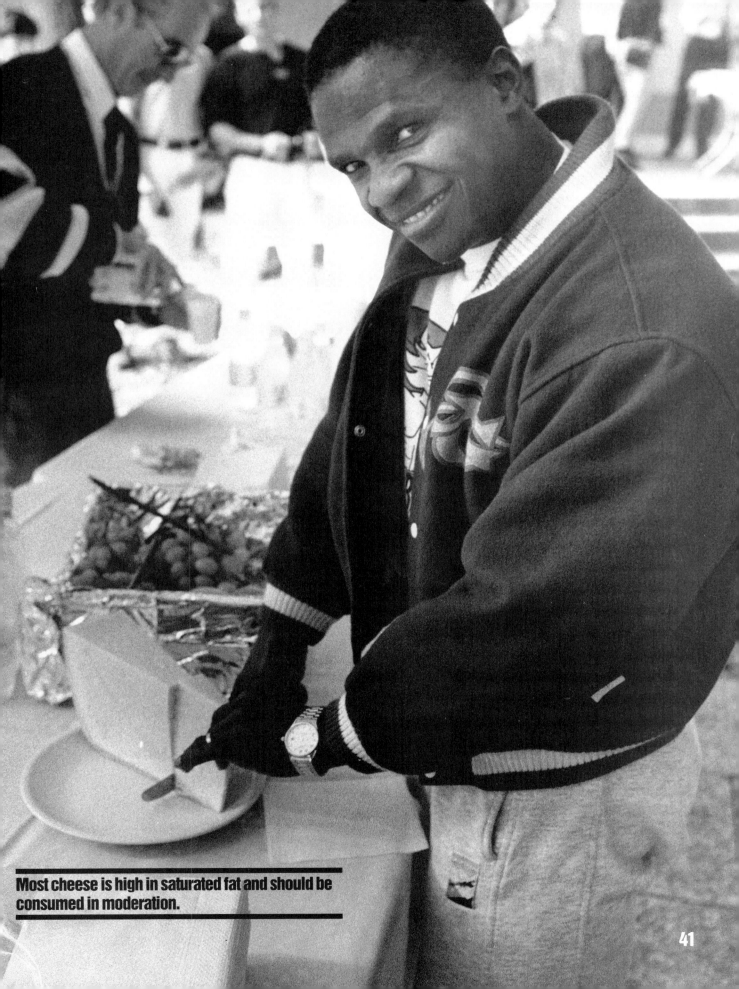

Most cheese is high in saturated fat and should be consumed in moderation.

BREAKFAST

Some of the best and worst foods in the American diet are consumed at breakfast. Such foods as bacon, sausage, butter, and cream cheese add considerable amounts of saturated fat to traditional breakfasts, while doughnuts, pastries, syrupy pancakes, and store-bought muffins add sugar, fat, and calories. Many cereals also provide hefty doses of sugar and sodium. And eggs, a staple of the American breakfast, supply one-third of all the cholesterol consumed in the United States. If your breakfast contains all the cholesterol or most of the sodium you should eat for the entire day, you may have trouble avoiding excesses later in the day.

It is probably easier to incorporate wholesome foods into your diet at breakfast than at other meals. Many low-fat, low-cholesterol, high-fiber foods are ideal morning fare, supplying nutrients that may be difficult to get in later meals.

The foods that supply a good breakfast—and suit most Americans' eating patterns—are some form of complex carbohydrates, such as breads and cereals. Also recommended is fruit or fruit juice high in vitamin C, and low-fat or skim milk or other dairy products. A small amount of fat helps provide satiety. Coffee or tea is harmless in moderation.

If you prefer chicken and vegetables, that's great. What people eat for breakfast is largely a cultural matter. But you should try to get fruit juice, whole grains, and milk products at lunch or dinner if you leave them out at breakfast.

LUNCH

For most people, lunch is a meal eaten hurriedly in the middle of a busy workday. As a result, people tend to choose foods that are quickly prepared and convenient to eat: a sandwich and a bag of chips from the local deli, a slice of pizza, or a fast-food burger and fries. Many of these foods, however, are high in fat and sodium and low in fiber. Fortunately, you don't have to give up convenience for health. Most traditional lunch fare can be modified to be more healthful.

At home and at restaurants, sandwiches are a standard lunch. But some of the old favorites—ham and Swiss, egg salad, and pastrami—may be dealing out more calories, cholesterol, and fat than most of us want to consume at one sitting. To create sandwiches that are more nutritious, follow these suggestions:

- Whole-grain breads give you more minerals and fiber than white breads or buns. Most bagels and pita breads are low in fat as well as sodium.

- Processed sandwich meats like bologna, salami, and liverwurst are usually high in saturated fat, cholesterol, and sodium. Roasting your own chicken or turkey for sandwiches is worth the effort. You'll cut down on calories, fat, and sodium. Discard all the visible fat on roast beef, ham, or pork.

- Instead of cheese or mayonnaise, add slices of vegetables or fruit to make a sandwich moister.

- A tasty, low-fat sandwich dressing can be made with plain, low-fat yogurt, or by blending equal parts of low-fat cottage cheese and buttermilk, flavored with herbs and spices. A tablespoon of such a mixture has only nine calories and a trace of fat.

- Catsup and prepared mustard are low-calorie, low-fat flavor boosters—10 to 24 calories per tablespoon—but they are high in sodium, with 150 to 180 milligrams per tablespoon. You can make sodium-free mustard by mixing mustard powder with water. Prepared horseradish has half the calories and one-tenth the sodium of mustard or catsup.

Besides sandwiches, another lunch possibility is the salad bar, a nutritious addition to many delis and restaurants. Still, you must choose wisely, since most salad bars are also stocked with numerous high-fat items.

The health-conscious, salad-bar diner should keep the following guidelines in mind:

- Choose your selections carefully. For the most part, stick to vegetables, fruits, and legumes. Cottage cheese can also be a good choice, provided it is the low-fat variety.

- Be aware that foods such as avocados, olives, sunflower seeds, bacon bits, cheese, and diced ham are high in fat and sometimes sodium. Use them sparingly. Think of such foods as condiments rather than the main focus of your salad.

- Avoid high-calorie salad dressings or limit the amount you use. A typical small ladle at the salad bar holds about two tablespoons of dressing. Two ladles of Italian, French, or blue cheese dressing contain approximately 300 calories, almost all of them from fat. Try using lemon juice, or vinegar mixed with a small amount of oil, or a low-calorie dressing instead.

- Predressed selections such as pasta or three-bean salad, marinated vegetables, and tuna salad are often doused with oil or mayonnaise. These items are also more likely to contain added sodium. Ask the management before you make a meal of any of them.

- Some salad bars offer hot foods as well. Many, such as macaroni and cheese, fried chicken, and meatballs, are unhealthy choices. Roast chicken or turkey would make a better addition to your salad. Soup can be another low-fat option if it is vegetable based, though it is likely to be high in sodium. Cream soups and those made with beef are often high in fat as well.

DINNER

For many people, dinner is the most important meal of the day. Research shows that Americans consume 42 to 45 percent of their total daily calories at dinner. The foods eaten at dinner contribute a significant amount of nutrients to the diet, but also a large proportion of the day's fat, cholesterol, and sodium.

It can be difficult to change eating habits at dinner, because that is the meal most

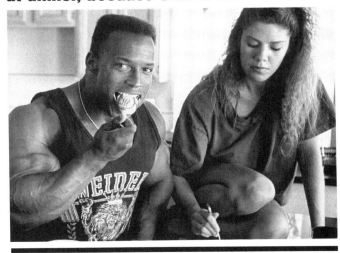

Almost all vegetables are low in calories.

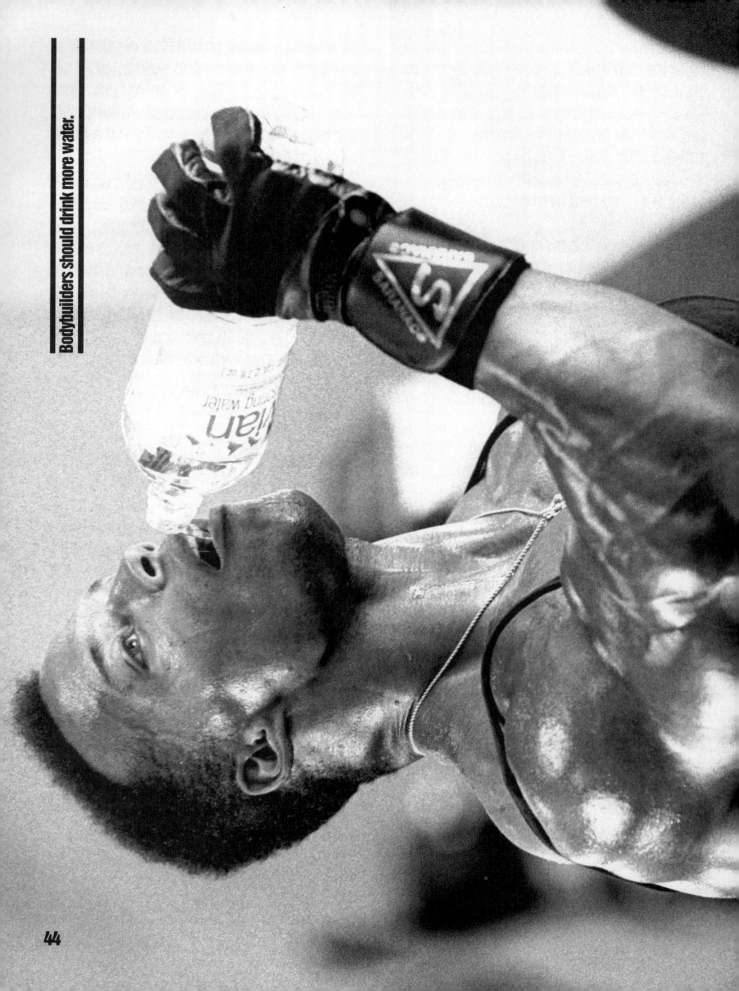

44

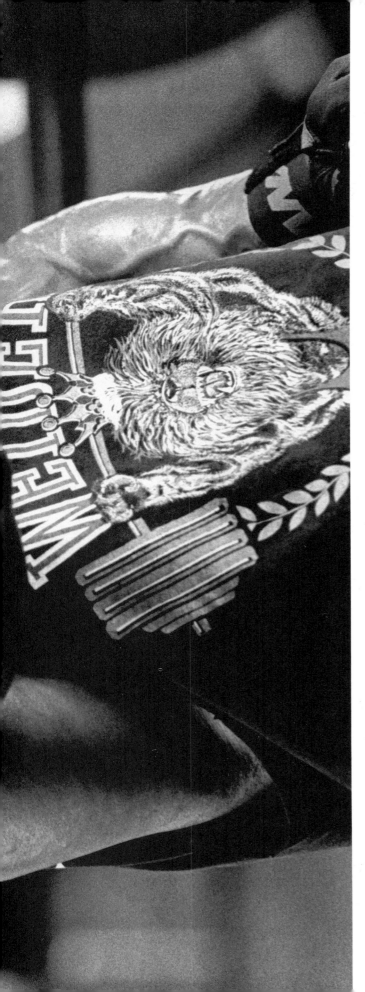

likely to be shared with other members of the household. One easy way to start is to make dinner a lighter meal. In fact, most nutritionists recommend that you spread your calories more evenly throughout the day. Creating a more healthy dinner doesn't mean you have to make drastic changes in the foods that you normally would eat. Here are some suggestions:

- Nutritious starters include raw vegetables—such as carrots, peppers, celery, and broccoli—with a dip made from low-fat yogurt, a green salad with low-fat dressing, or a chicken-based soup.

- Brown rice instead of white adds potassium, phosphorus, and fiber to your meal.

- Other healthful side dishes include steamed vegetables, grains such as wheat pilaf, baked potatoes topped with salsa or low-fat yogurt, and legumes flavored with herbs and spices.

- A steady diet of dinners centering around red meat can contribute more fat, cholesterol, and protein than is healthy. Fortunately, there are many alternatives, such as white-meat chicken or fish.

- Traditional desserts such as cakes, pies, custards, and ice creams are high in fat and should be consumed in moderation. Better choices are fresh fruit, frozen yogurt, ice milk, and sherbet.

GROWTH AND HEALTH

With the understanding and appreciation of the steps to healthy eating in this chapter, you can be sure that your body will have all the essential nutrients it needs for maximum growth. Furthermore, you will also possess all the health and well-being that good nutrition can bring.

CHAPTER 4
GENETICS: ONE IN A MILLION

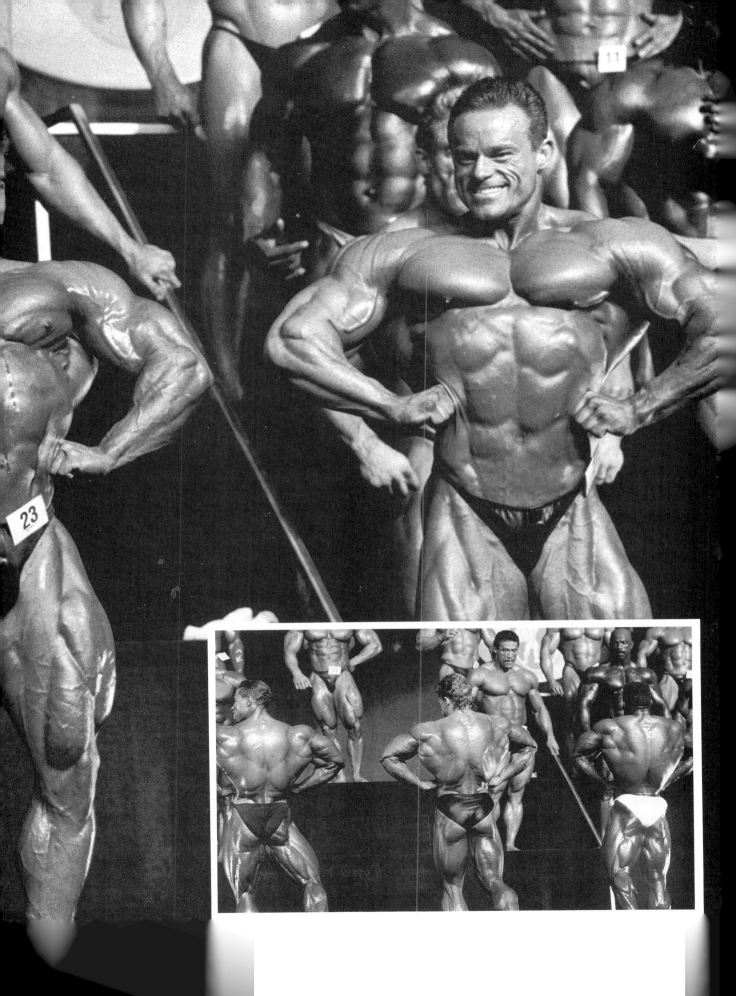

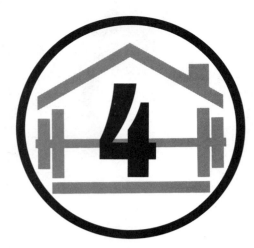

Suppose for a few minutes that one of your foremost goals in life is to be very tall, say six feet ten inches, or even seven feet. This is an especially far-reaching goal, since you are only five feet eight inches tall. Also suppose that you have never heard of basketball and never seen a basketball game.

HEIGHT AND
PROFESSIONAL BASKETBALL

Then, one day while you are visiting a large city such as Los Angeles, Atlanta, or New York, you attend a professional basketball game for the first time.

"Wow," you exclaim after the initial quarter, "I've never in my life seen so many tall men in one place." You've just got to get down close to the court for a better look. Sure enough, when you are near the court, perhaps only a few yards from some of the players, you are convinced that your long-desired goal can be obtained.

How? Simply by becoming skilled at bouncing and shooting a basketball. Almost anyone should be able to see the relationship.

When you return home, the first thing you do is go to your local sporting goods store and purchase a basketball, a backboard, and a basket. Then you round up every basketball book you can find from your library and bookstore. With a lot of practice, you figure, you'll start growing taller in no time.

So you begin practicing. And you continue on a daily basis—for weeks and months.

Unfortunately, you don't get taller. The only thing that increases is your proficiency at dribbling and shooting. Nothing you seem to do with the ball makes you taller. But why were all the players on the professional basketball teams so tall?

You decide to seek out a basketball coach and ask him what your problem is. Much to your surprise, the coach explains to you that playing basketball has no effect on your height. You must have the genes to get taller, the coach says, and if you do, you will get taller whether or not you play basketball.

To play professional basketball, an individual must be very tall. He must learn the skills of basketball at a young age. This is not to say, however, that most people cannot learn the skills of basketball and enjoy playing the game. But there is little chance for an individual to play professional basketball unless he has inherited genes that make him tall.

So far, so good. You should now definitely see the connection among genetics, being very tall, and playing professional basketball.

LARGE MUSCLES AND
THE MR. OLYMPIA

Now I want you to suppose that your goal is to have very large muscles. Also, I want you to suppose that you've never heard of bodybuilding and never seen a bodybuilding contest.

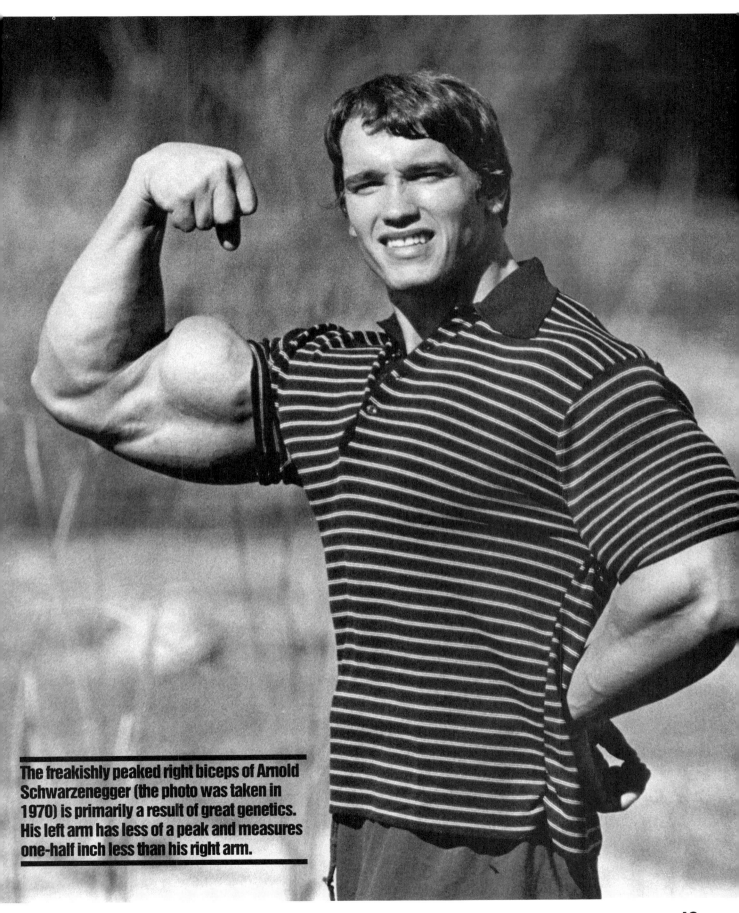

The freakishly peaked right biceps of Arnold Schwarzenegger (the photo was taken in 1970) is primarily a result of great genetics. His left arm has less of a peak and measures one-half inch less than his right arm.

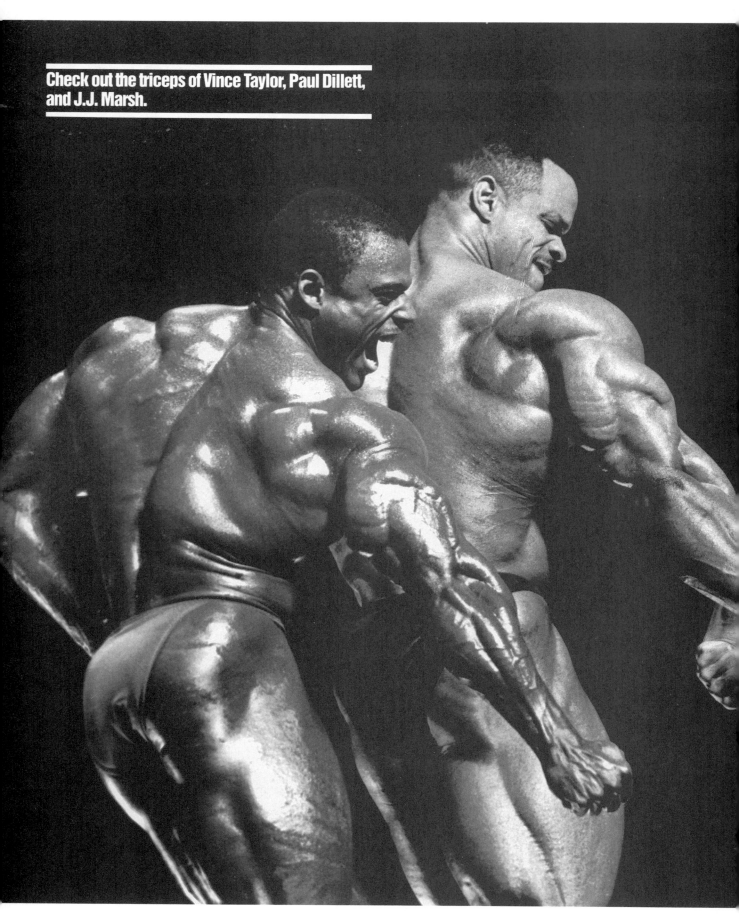

Check out the triceps of Vince Taylor, Paul Dillett, and J.J. Marsh.

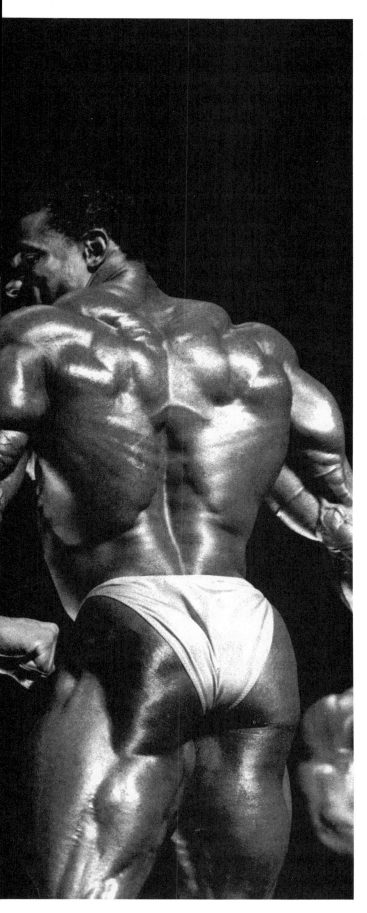

Then one day you attend the Mr. Olympia contest and sit in the front row. Furthermore, you get to go backstage at intermission and watch the finalists pump up. You are simply awed by the size of these guys.

You can't help but notice that all of these bodybuilders are lifting weights backstage. Lifting weights, you reason, must be the secret to getting very large muscles.

So the next day you purchase some weights, buy some bodybuilding books, and start training. Months and years go by, and yes, you get bigger and stronger, but you don't look anything like Dorian Yates, Lee Haney, Arnold Schwarzenegger, or whoever your hero is. What are you doing wrong? What's the answer? You decide to ask a coach or an expert.

THE DIFFERENCE BETWEEN BASKET-BALL AND BODYBUILDING COACHES

Here's where the two stories differ. The average basketball coach understands the importance of genetics in his sport. The average bodybuilding coach doesn't. The bodybuilding coach is likely to tell you that you need more training, different exercises, or additional food supplements. He is not likely to tell you that you must have unusual genetics to get unusually large muscles. Professional bodybuilders have inherited muscular characteristics that make them unique.

In fact, the men who enter the Mr. Olympia are as unusual as the men who are seven feet tall and play professional basketball. Both are giants: giants in muscle or giants in height.

In my opinion, approximately one in a million men in the United States has the genetic potential to be seven feet tall, or the genetic potential to build excessively large Mr. Olympia-type muscles. <u>One in a million:</u> think about it!

Let's take a closer look at genetic potential and muscle building.

INHERITED CHARACTERISTICS

At least seven inherited characteristics influence your bodybuilding capacity. Here's a brief examination of each factor:

- <u>Muscle length.</u> The length of your muscle bellies is the single most important factor in determining potential size. Your muscles attach to bones by tendons. If you surgically removed an entire muscle from your body with the tendons intact, you'd notice that the tendons at either end are composed of very dense tissue. Follow this dense tissue until it tapers into the muscle. Now cut the tendons off at either end. What you're left with is called the muscle belly, the meaty part of the tissue. The longer a muscle belly, the greater the cross-sectional area and volume can become. Those with huge muscles, or the potential for developing them, have short tendons and long muscle bellies. For a muscle to be wide, it must be exceptionally long. An exceptionally long muscle doesn't have to be wide, but it has the potential to be and it responds quickly to proper training. More details will follow.

- <u>Muscle fiber type.</u> As stated previously, individual muscle fibers basically have either slow-twitch or fast-twitch characteristics. It is to your advantage to have mostly fast-twitch muscle fibers throughout your body, since they have greater potential for size.

- <u>Tendon insertion point.</u> Where a tendon attaches to the bone is called the tendon insertion point. The tendon insertion point can greatly influence your strength output and overall training effect. For example, your biceps tendon crosses the front side of your elbow and attaches to your lower arm bone near the elbow joint. Let's say for discussion purposes that the tendon attaches exactly one inch from the joint. If, however, we could move the insertion point a quarter inch farther away from the elbow joint, would that be an advantage or disadvantage in building muscle? It would be a great advantage, because it would dramatically improve your leverage. Greater leverage would mean greater strength. Greater strength would mean you'd be able to lift heavier weights. Lifting heavier weights would produce more growth stimulation.

- <u>Body proportions.</u> Height, torso length, shoulder and hip width, and length of arms and legs are crucial determinants of an individual's appearance as well as his ability to perform. In a bodybuilding competition, it helps to have broad shoulders, narrow hips, a short torso, medium-length arms, and long legs. Arnold Schwarzenegger has such proportions. A power lifter, on the other hand, is aided by having narrow shoulders, wide hips, a long torso, long arms, and short legs.

- <u>Skeletal formation.</u> A competitive bodybuilder must have bones that are large

The left flexed arm of Ray Mentzer measured 20 3/8 inches when this photo was taken on July 9, 1983. Notice the fullness of his triceps—a result of an extremely long triceps muscle.

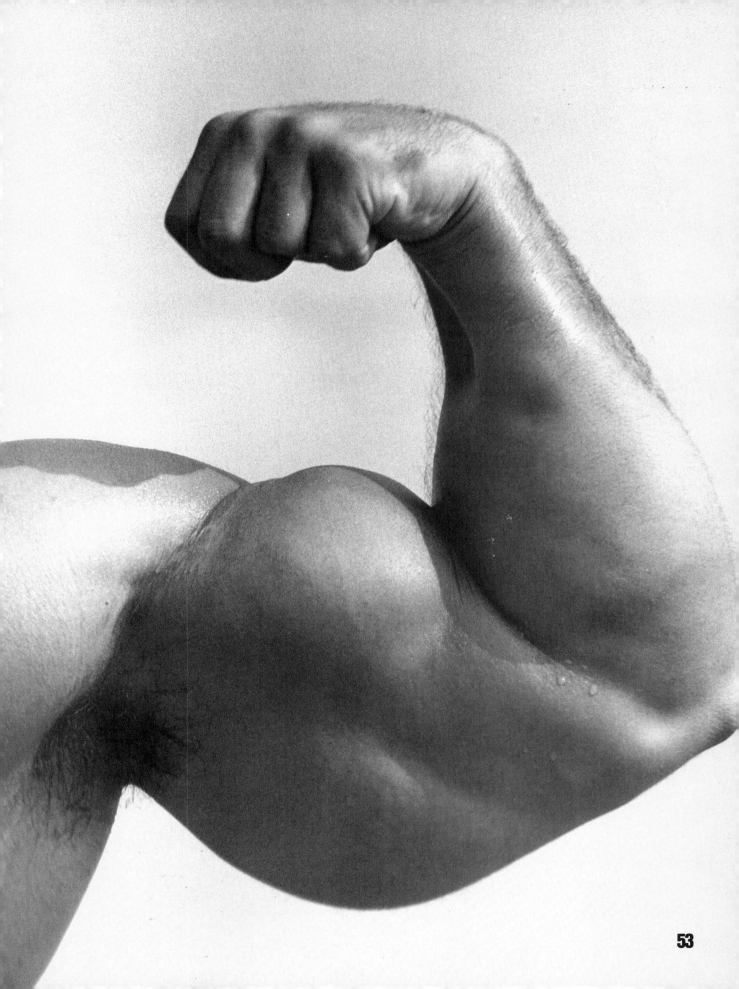

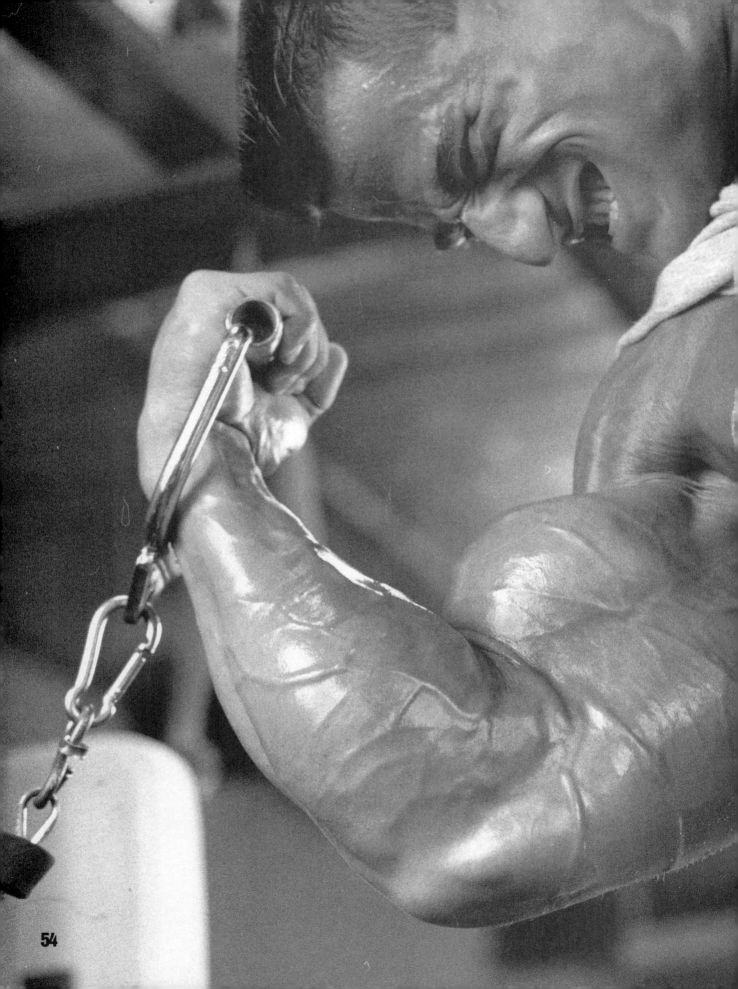

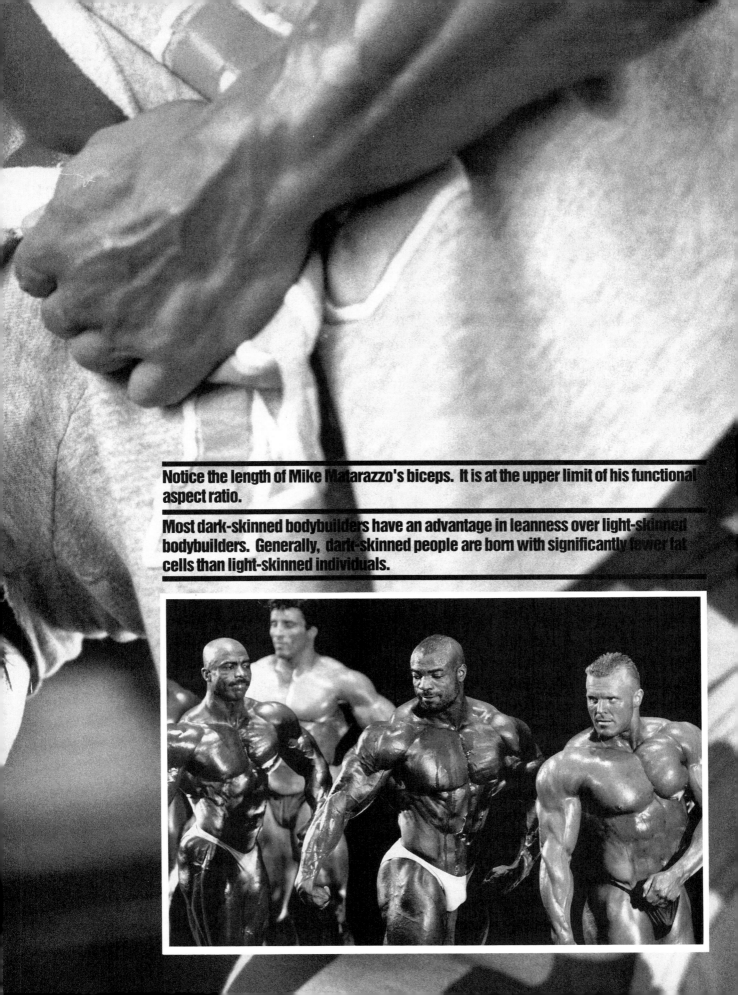

Notice the length of Mike Matarazzo's biceps. It is at the upper limit of his functional aspect ratio.

Most dark-skinned bodybuilders have an advantage in leanness over light-skinned bodybuilders. Generally, dark-skinned people are born with significantly fewer fat cells than light-skinned individuals.

enough to support heavy musculature. But his bones, especially at the joints, must not exceed a certain size, or he may lose the necessary aesthetic qualities contingent on bone structure.

- Body fat. Most nutrition authorities believe that the number of fat cells you have is determined genetically. Research reveals that total fat-cell numbers can vary as much as tenfold among individuals. Fat thicknesses also are inherited in the same way as height, muscle lengths, and nose shapes. Obviously, great muscular definition requires that an individual have a small number of body-fat cells and that he store most of his fat around his internal organs and not directly under his skin.

- Skin color. Generally, bodybuilders with dark skin, hair, and eyes—compared to those with light skin, blond hair, and blue eyes—have a genetic advantage where body leanness and extreme muscular definition are concerned. Why is this generalization true? Because there exists a strong relationship between fat-cell numbers and the annual mean temperature of where a person's ancestors came from. The colder the mean temperature, the greater the cell numbers and the fatter the people. The warmer the mean temperature, the leaner the people. Cold climates also reinforced light skin and hair, because such individuals were able to extract more vitamin D from sunlight than persons with dark skin were. Warm, tropical environments, on the other hand, were better suited for dark-skinned people. Fair-skinned individuals do not adjust well to hot, sunny climates. Today, scientists can document the extraordinary degree to which our physical condition still is programmed by blueprints laid down by our ancestors from thousands of years ago.

MORE ABOUT MUSCLE LENGTH

Muscle length, muscle-fiber type, tendon insertion point, body proportions, skeletal formation, body fat, and skin color are important to your bodybuilding success. What you are born with in these areas is what you die with. You can do little or nothing to affect them in a positive manner. You can, however, understand each of these factors and use each to explore your bodybuilding potential in a realistic manner.

The most instrumental factor in your quest for muscular size remains muscle length. While simple in theory, the muscle-length connection is still widely ignored. I remember the first time I heard Arthur Jones discuss it in 1973. Jones used the concept of aspect ratio to make it clear. Aspect ratio deals with the relationship between an object's length and width.

For example, framed pictures that you hang on the wall have an established width-to-height ratio that is pleasing to the eye. The standard five-by-seven-inch or eight-by-ten-inch photograph falls under this category. Vary significantly from this aspect ratio and the picture doesn't look right—it doesn't work, it doesn't function correctly.

That same aspect ratio, Jones reasoned, applies to muscles. For a muscle to function, it must contract or shorten. During contraction, the thin actin filaments with the involved muscle fibers are pulled toward the thick myosin filaments. What happens is similar to interlacing your fingertips and

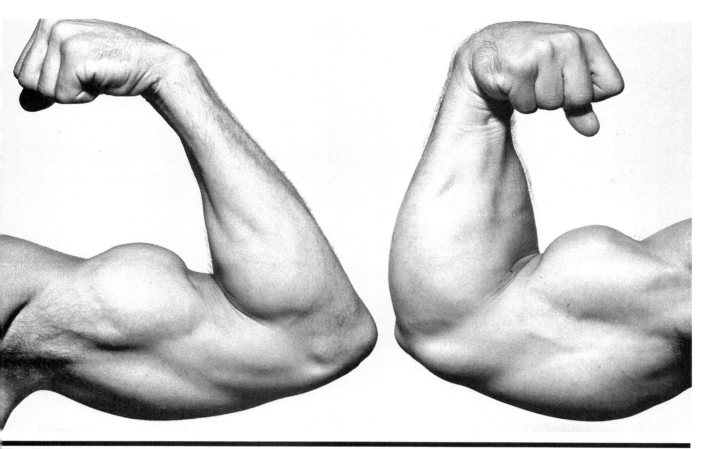

The difference between average and great biceps potential is shown in this comparison. The arm on the left is actually bent too much. The left forearm should be perpendicular to the upper arm bone, in a similar fashion to the arm on the right. Nevertheless, the gaps between the biceps and forearms are plainly evident. You could fit two fingers into the gap on the left and less than one finger in the space on the right. The left arm has average to good potential, while the right arm has great potential.

smoothly pushing them together and then pulling them apart. Since most muscles have a tear-drop-like shape, as the fibers enlarge, the angle of pull on the tendon becomes less and less direct. Past a certain size, the muscle—or at least part of it—would fail to contract. It simply would not function. Its aspect ratio would not allow it to work.

In other words, a short muscle cannot be very wide because its angle of pull would be so poor that it would not be able to contract efficiently. The body, therefore, would not allow a short, wide muscle to develop.

To function effectively, a wide muscle must be long. And the length of your muscles is 100 percent genetically determined. You cannot lengthen them through exercise, nutrition, drugs, or anything else.

The most easily measured muscle lengths are the biceps and triceps of the upper arms, the flexors of the forearms, and the gastrocnemius of the calves. Several tests to determine muscle length and potential are described on pages 82 - 84 of my book <u>100 High-Intensity Ways to Improve Your Bodybuilding</u> (Perigee Books, 1989).

A SIMPLE TEST FOR BICEPS LENGTH

Dr. Wayne Westcott, strength-training consultant for the national YMCA, has designed a lay version of my biceps potential test. Here's what you need to do.

Take off your shirt and hit a biceps pose with your best arm in front of a mirror. Make sure your hand is fully supinated, or twisted outward, which accentuates the peak on your biceps. The bend in your arm, or the angle between the bones in your upper arm and forearm, should be ninety degrees.

Now look at the gap between your contracted biceps and forearm. How wide is the gap?

To find out, see how many fingers from your other hand you can fit into the gap. Flatten out your fingers and give it a try. Remember to keep the bend in your flexed arm at ninety degrees.

If you can get three fingers in the space, then your biceps length is below average and your potential is poor. Two fingers mean average length and average potential. One finger in the gap signals above-average muscle length and good potential. If you are unable to squeeze one finger in the space, then you have exceptional biceps muscles and your potential is great.

THE LONG AND SHORT OF IT

If you have a short biceps, it does not mean that all your major muscles are short. Differences exist in the same person from one side of the body to the other and from one body part to another. It is a rare individual who has uniform potential over the entire body. Often we see a bodybuilder who has great arms and legs but a weak torso. Then there is the athlete with large thighs and small calves; this is most prevalent among blacks. For reasons unknown, most blacks inherit short gastrocnemius muscles and long tendons in their lower legs.

Examples of current bodybuilders with long muscle bellies in certain body parts are as follows:

- Biceps:
  Mike Matarazzo, Vince Taylor, Paul Dillett
- Triceps:
  Thierry Pastel, Shawn Ray, Kevin Levrone
- Quadriceps:
  Paul DeMayo, Kevin Levrone
- Hamstrings:
  Shawn Ray, Flex Wheeler
- Latissimus dorsi:
  Lee Haney, Dorian Yates
- Gastrocnemius:
  Mike Matarazzo, Vince Taylor

Even though you may not be blessed with the muscle-belly lengths of Paul Dillett or Kevin Levrone, you can still grow bigger and stronger. Make an intelligent effort, however, to be realistic. Whatever your potential, the principles in this book will get you to your limits in the most efficient manner.

Both Paul DeMayo and Denise Rutkowski have long muscles throughout their bodies.

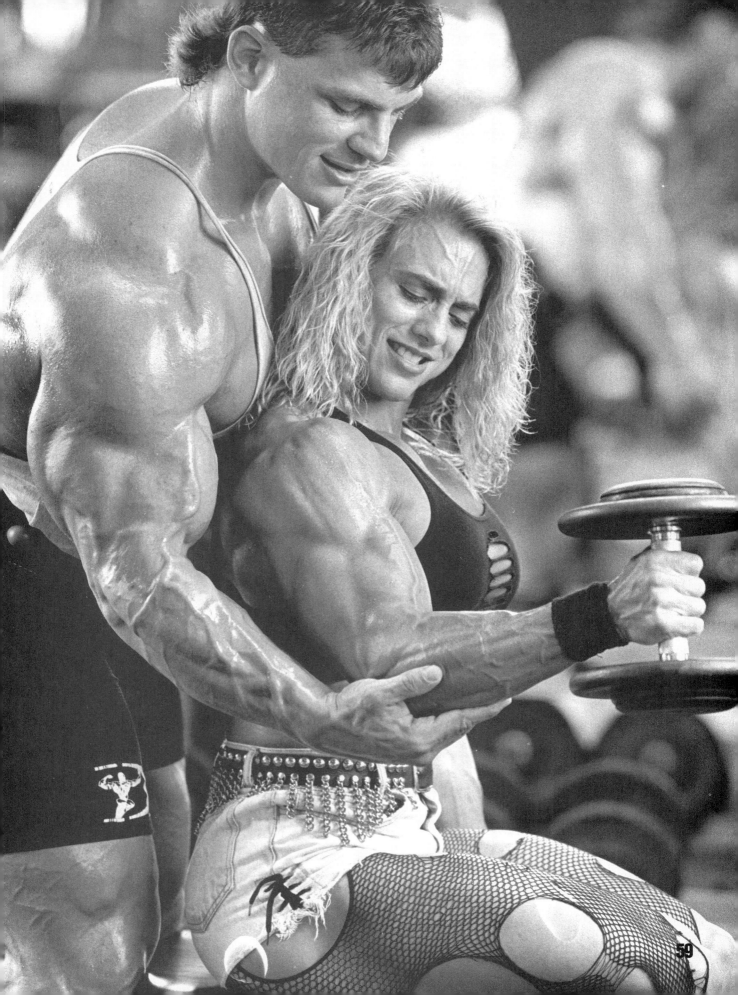

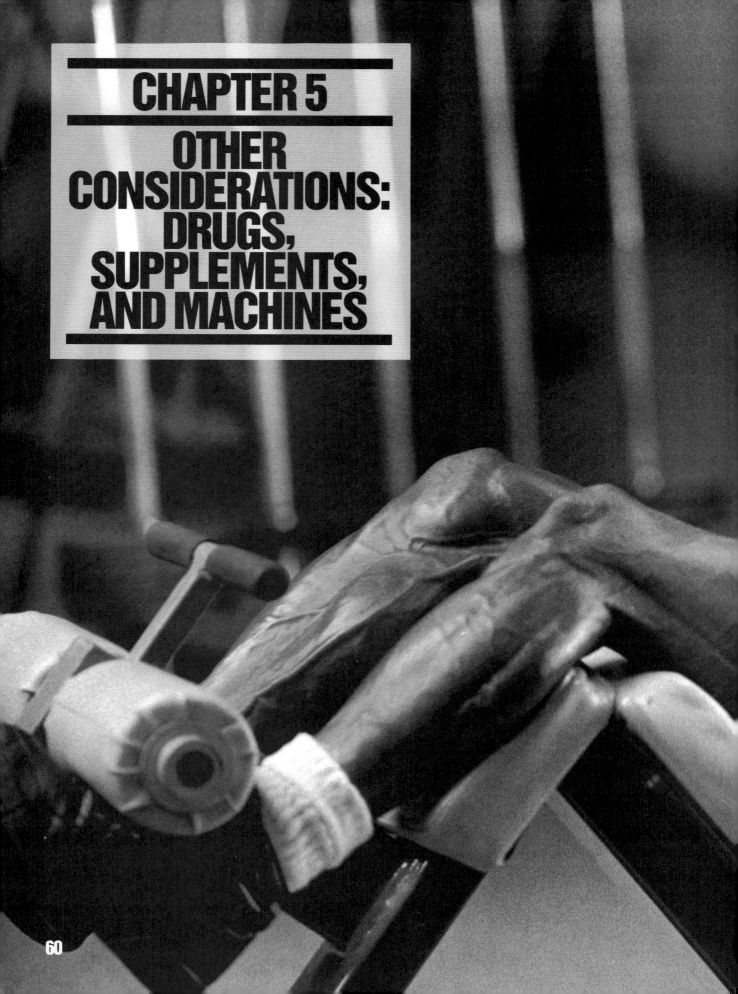

CHAPTER 5

OTHER CONSIDERATIONS: DRUGS, SUPPLEMENTS, AND MACHINES

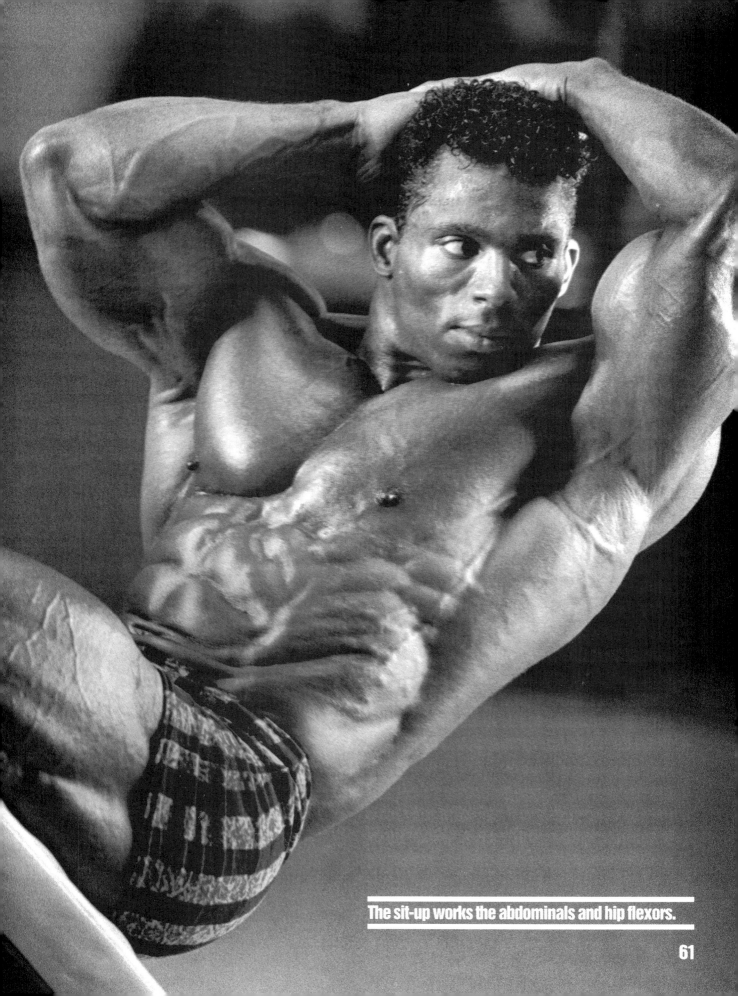

The sit-up works the abdominals and hip flexors.

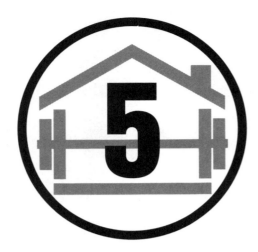

5

More than any other sport or fitness endeavor, bodybuilding success (especially at the competitive level) is based on having the right genetic potential.

Yes, proper training will make your muscles bigger and stronger, and it will do so quickly. But no, proper training will not make your muscles freakishly large, unless your muscles are unusually long to begin with. The one-in-a-million probability of having the necessary muscle lengths doesn't help your chances either, does it?

Hope reigns eternal, however, with most bodybuilders. Where there's a will, there's a way, goes the old saying. If you believe what's stated as fact in the muscle magazines, as well as the "newly discovered secrets" of mail-order entrepreneurs, then almost any would-be bodybuilder can eventually look like his favorite Mr. Olympia contestant. The key, supposedly, is the right combination of drugs, food supplements, and equipment or machines.

Let's examine each one.

DRUGS

If you're a reader of bodybuilding magazines, I'm sure you were saddened by the death of Mohammad Benaziza. Mohammad was a professional bodybuilder who died shortly after he was declared the winner of the IFBB Dutch Grand Prix in Rotterdam, Holland, on October 3, 1992.

What killed Mohammad? Reports indicate that this thirty-three-year-old bodybuilder, who was at the height of his career, died from a combination of many things working against him. A primary factor, according to Greg Zulak of <u>Musclemag International</u> (March 1993), was drugs, drugs, and more drugs!

Here's what the reports revealed:

- Benaziza was taking high dosages of diuretics (Lasix and Aldactone, both strong prescription drugs) prior to the contest to rid his body of excess fluids.

- Benaziza had stopped drinking all fluids for three days before the competition.

- Benaziza was a heavy user of steroids, growth hormones, clenbuterol, and other so-called anabolic agents. He was described as a "walking drugstore" by one competitor.

- Benaziza, according to the article by Greg Zulak, had been arrested in France earlier in the year for importing and selling steroids.

Why was Mohammad taking so many drugs? Probably because in his mind, they offered him hope, hope of being Mr. Olympia. At five feet two inches tall, Mohammad was borderline too short to win the top prize in bodybuilding. If everything was equal bodywise except height, the taller man would always win. Benaziza

Daryl Stafford has great abdominals and hip flexors.

62

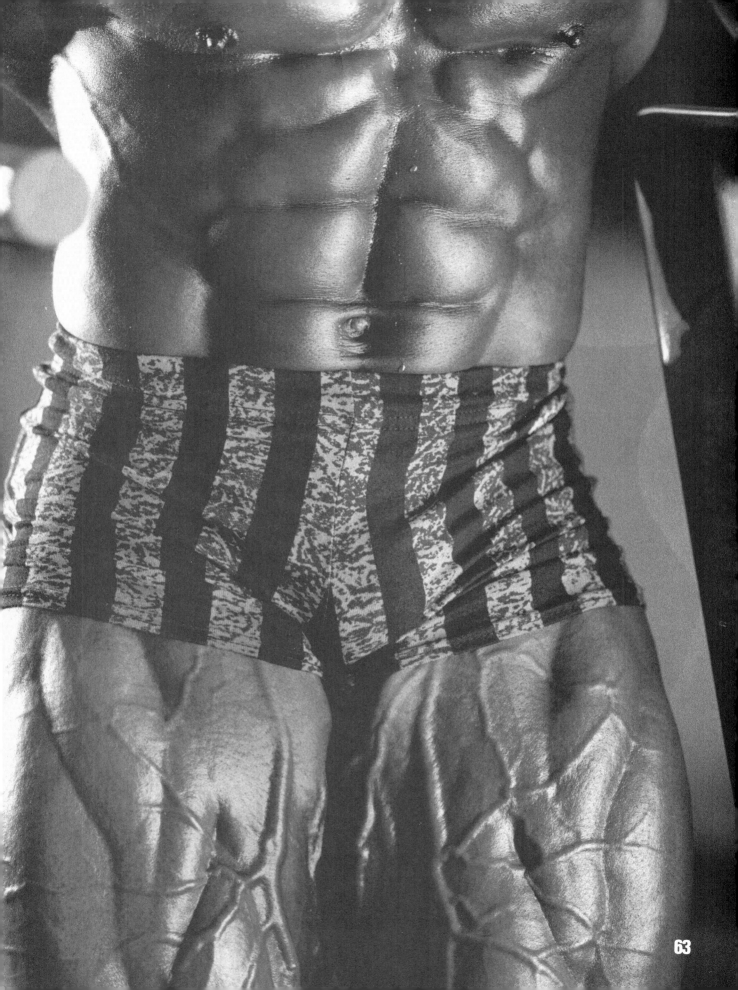

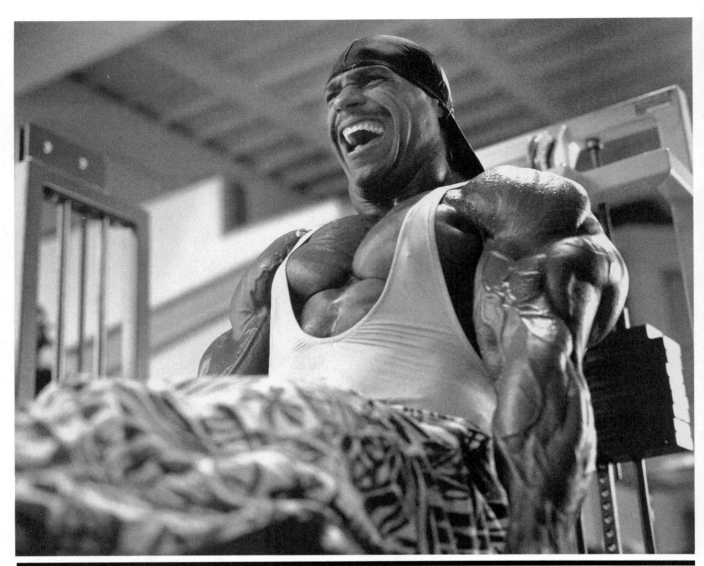

Look at the unusual size and shape of Mike Christian's left triceps.

would have to be significantly better than a taller man to win.

That was Mohammad's goal: to be significantly better than his taller competitors. "That's why he took everything to the extreme," said one of his close friends, "and it killed him!"

MILLIONS ON STEROIDS

"Between two and three million Americans are currently using anabolic steroids," according to Bill Phillips, editor of Muscle Media 2000 magazine. But why, especially when there's a long list of potential life-threatening risks and altered psychological behaviors associated with steroids? Furthermore, it is now a felony not only to use or possess steroids but to encourage someone to do so. For the most part, it is illegal for physicians to prescribe steroids.

As a result, Bill Phillips now estimates that most of what is being sold as steroids in this country are counterfeit. Unscrupulous people attain a sample of the legitimate product. Then they have the label, box, and insert reprinted. Glass vials and small bottles are easy to purchase. As for what goes into these products, 90 percent of the contents contain no steroid ingredients at all. Most counterfeit versions of injectable steroids are only vegetable oil. Most tablets are fillers like potassium and calcium. Many are packaged under unsanitary conditions.

But even so, the demand for steroids is still prevalent. In fact, it seems to be increasing.

SAY NO TO DRUGS

It is our American performance-oriented, appeanace-oriented, instant-gratification-oriented, and most of all, drug-oriented society that is to blame. Almost all of us—old, young, and in between—are partially at fault.

You can do your part by refusing to take drugs in connection with your bodybuilding.

Say NO now. And continue to say NO.

Say YES to proper exercise, adequate rest, and good nutrition.

FOOD SUPPLEMENTS

Food supplements are usually defined as concentrated nutrients that are available in liquids, powders, pills, or tablets. They are sold throughout the United States in health-food stores, fitness centers, pharmacies, supermarkets, and through the mail. One of the largest buyers of food supplements are bodybuilders. Most of the advertisements in any muscle magazine are for supplements.

Here are headlines from some recent advertisements:

- **Experience Mind-Blowing Gains with the World's #1 Mass Builder**

- **Forge Your Body with the Most Powerful Bodybuilding Formula Ever**
- **100% Guaranteed Anabolic Muscle-Building Steroids Replacement**
- **Energy Explosion: A Blast of Unrelenting Power for Longer Workouts !**
- **Want Really Hard Muscles? Fuel Inject with Vanadyl Sulfate**
- **Extraordinary Results Require an Extraordinary Protein**
- **Nitrogen Retention/Anti-Catabolic Formula**
- **Plutonium Power Pump**
- **The Anabolic Igniter Flex Fire!**
- **Explosive Workout Stack System**

The headlines are for products that can be grouped under four categories: weight gainers/energy producers, protein supplements, vitamin-mineral pills, and steroid replacements. Let's examine each one.

WEIGHT GAINERS /
ENERGY PRODUCERS

Most of these products are calorie-rich powders that come in various flavors, such as chocolate, vanilla, and banana. The nutrient breakdown is usually predominantly carbohydrates and moderate amounts of proteins and fats. Often these products contain vitamins and minerals. When mixed with milk they make a tasty shake.

All of the essential ingredients in any of these powders can be found in the standard foods that compose a balanced diet. Most of these powders are fortified with nonessential substances that cause the products to be more expensive.

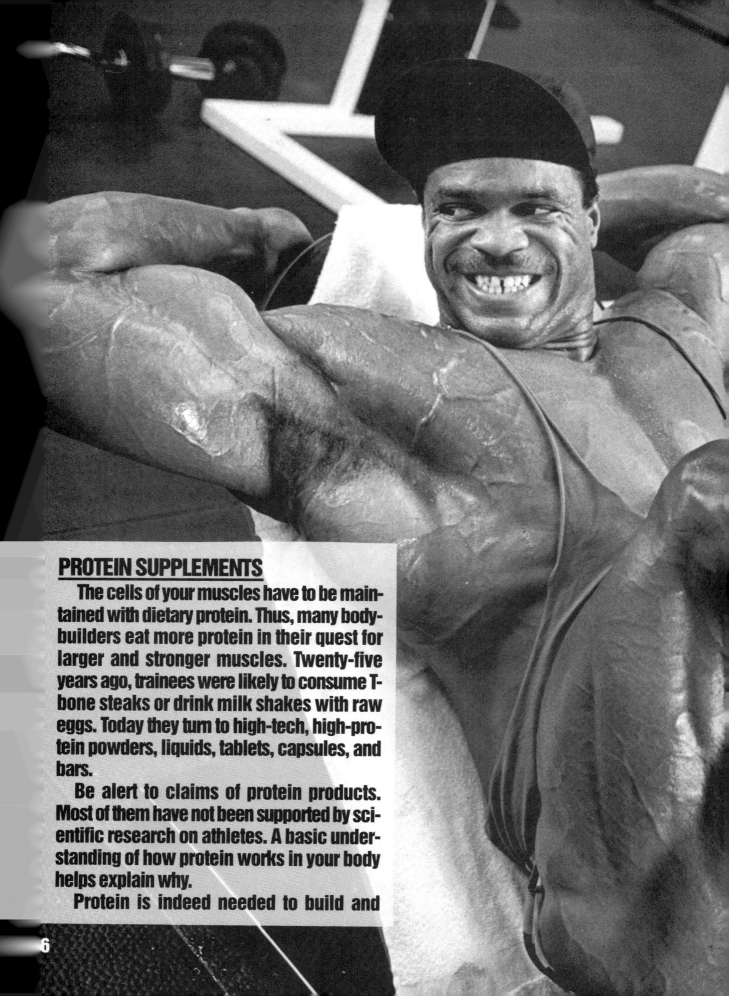

PROTEIN SUPPLEMENTS

The cells of your muscles have to be maintained with dietary protein. Thus, many bodybuilders eat more protein in their quest for larger and stronger muscles. Twenty-five years ago, trainees were likely to consume T-bone steaks or drink milk shakes with raw eggs. Today they turn to high-tech, high-protein powders, liquids, tablets, capsules, and bars.

Be alert to claims of protein products. Most of them have not been supported by scientific research on athletes. A basic understanding of how protein works in your body helps explain why.

Protein is indeed needed to build and

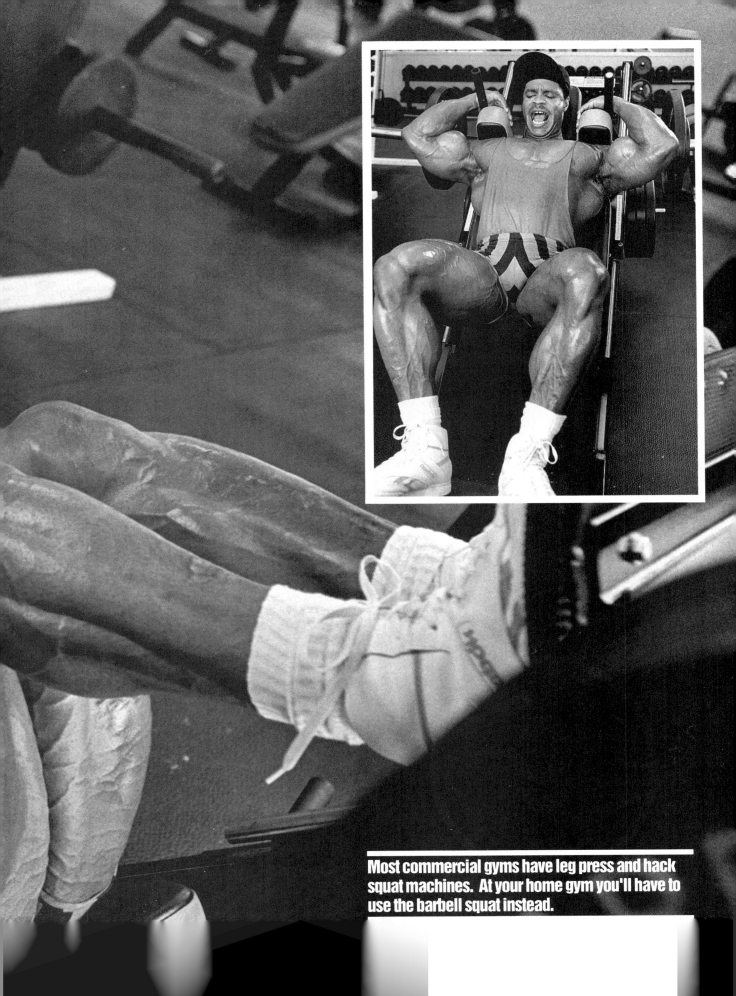

Most commercial gyms have leg press and hack squat machines. At your home gym you'll have to use the barbell squat instead.

maintain not only muscles but all cells in your body. But consuming more protein won't by itself stimulate muscular growth. Excess protein simply breaks down in your body and is burned for energy or, if not used, is converted to fat.

Some supplements have their isolated amino acids touted as being better absorbed by your body than whole protein. Healthy individuals, however, have no problem digesting and absorbing the amino acids from whole protein. Consuming large quantities of isolated amino acids is not advised, since your body needs a balanced mixture of amino acids to synthesize protein. The excessive intake of a single amino acid may interfere with the absorption of other amino acids and as a result inhibit protein synthesis.

How much protein does a young bodybuilder require each day? Probably a lot less than you think.

The Recommended Dietary Allowance for protein is .36 grams per pound of body weight. Thus, if you weighed 180 pounds, you would need 64.8 grams of protein per day. Most bodybuilders consume that much protein per meal, or over 200 grams a day, and that doesn't include another 100 grams per day from supplements.

Such massive protein intakes are completely unnecessary for muscular growth. In fact, excessive dietary protein over extended periods can seriously damage your liver and kidneys.

VITAMIN-MINERAL PILLS

Bodybuilders rarely need vitamin-mineral supplements. Taking extra vitamins and minerals will not speed up the muscle-building process, despite all the claims. The continuing hoopla over vitamin-mineral supplements has inspired thousands of careful scientific studies, and in almost every case researchers have found that these nutrients simply cannot perform the miracles that some people say they will.

Furthermore, megadoses of vitamins are not only wasteful, they are potentially hazardous. Relying on pills makes it easy to far exceed recommended levels, whereas it's almost impossible to reach megadose levels if you get your vitamins through the foods you eat.

STEROID REPLACEMENTS

Many new food supplements are being marketed as "steroid replacements" or "natural steroids." The ingredients in these products are not the same as steroids. Such compounds as vanadyl sulfate, chromium picolinate, yohimbe bark, ginseng, and bee pollen may sound interesting, but their effect is minimal. Save your money for something of real value.

WEIGHT-TRAINING MACHINES

Twenty years ago, only a few companies manufactured muscle-building machines. Universal manufactured a multistation machine that simulated basic barbell exercise. And Nautilus was just starting to make its heavy-duty machines with cams that varied the resistance. Today there are over forty different companies that sell various weight-training equipment.

Most of these machines can be grouped according to five categories:

- Multistation weight-stack machines
- Single-station weight-stack machines
- Single-station plate-loading machines

- Isokinetic machines
- Computerized machines

How many of these machines are practical for consideration in your home gym? Not many, unless money and space are not an issue.

The multistation weight-stack machines basically make barbell exercises safer and more convenient to load and unload. The larger units, such as those manufactured by Universal, are well made and expensive. The smaller units, which are sold via mail order, are too flimsy for heavy-duty use.

Single-station weight-stack machines, such as those made famous by Nautilus, are well made, expensive, and different from some traditional barbell exercises. Machines such as the pullover, leg extension, and leg curl provide direct resistance for the lats, quadriceps, and hamstrings—something you can't do with a barbell.

Single-station plate-loading machines are approximately half the price of weight-stack machines. You have to provide your own weight plates, and usually these weights have to be Olympic style with the larger holes. Nautilus and Hammer manufacture excellent machines of this type.

Isokinetic machines do not have weight stacks. Resistance is supplied by some form of friction: mechanical or liquid. Usually because of the nature of the isokinetic overload, there is no negative resistance. Isokinetic machines would be of limited value in a home gym.

Computerized machines, such as Cybex and MedX, are very expensive. They are used mostly in a testing and rehabilitation setting. Other computerized training machines, such as Life Fitness, are made for large fitness centers. None of the computerized machines would be practical for a home gym.

THE SAFE, EFFICIENT WAY

The least expensive and most practical home-gym exercise tool remains the barbell. When the basic exercises that are described in this book are applied intensely, and combined with adequate rest and nutritious food, you can reach your genetic potential safely and efficiently. And you can do so without life-threatening drugs, without food supplements, and without expensive machines.

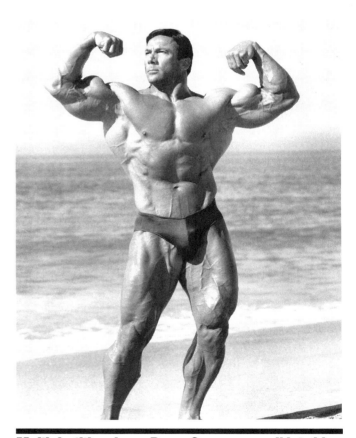

Multiple-title winner Boyer Coe, now well into his forties, trains on a combination of machines and free weights. When he was a teenager, however, Boyer got his start by exercising in a home gym with barbells and dumbbells.

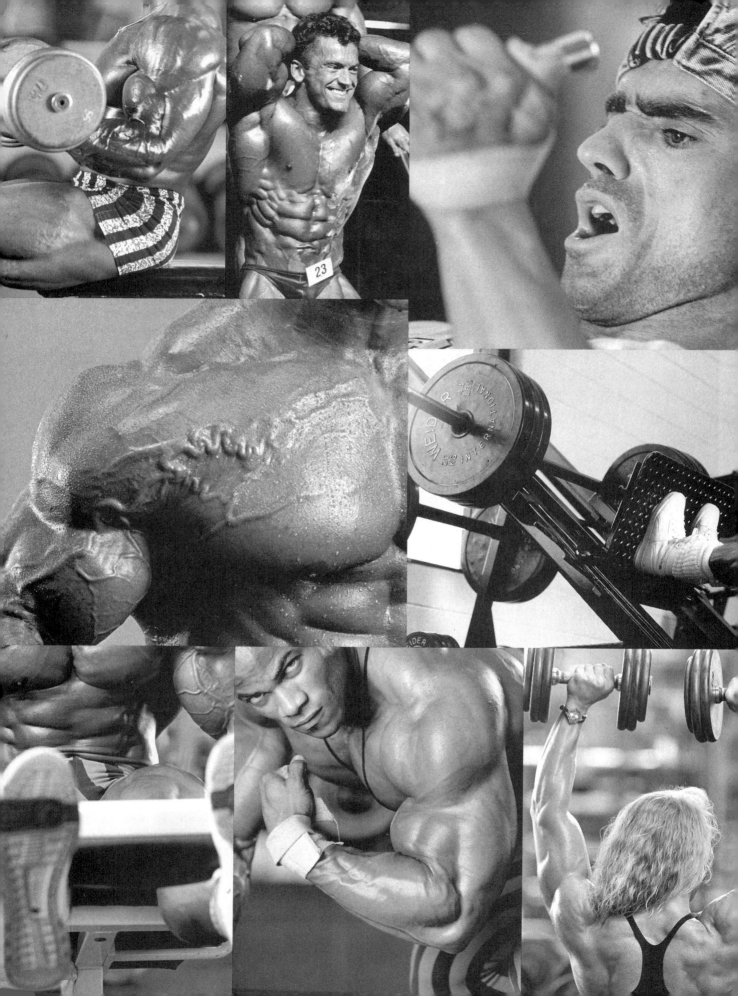

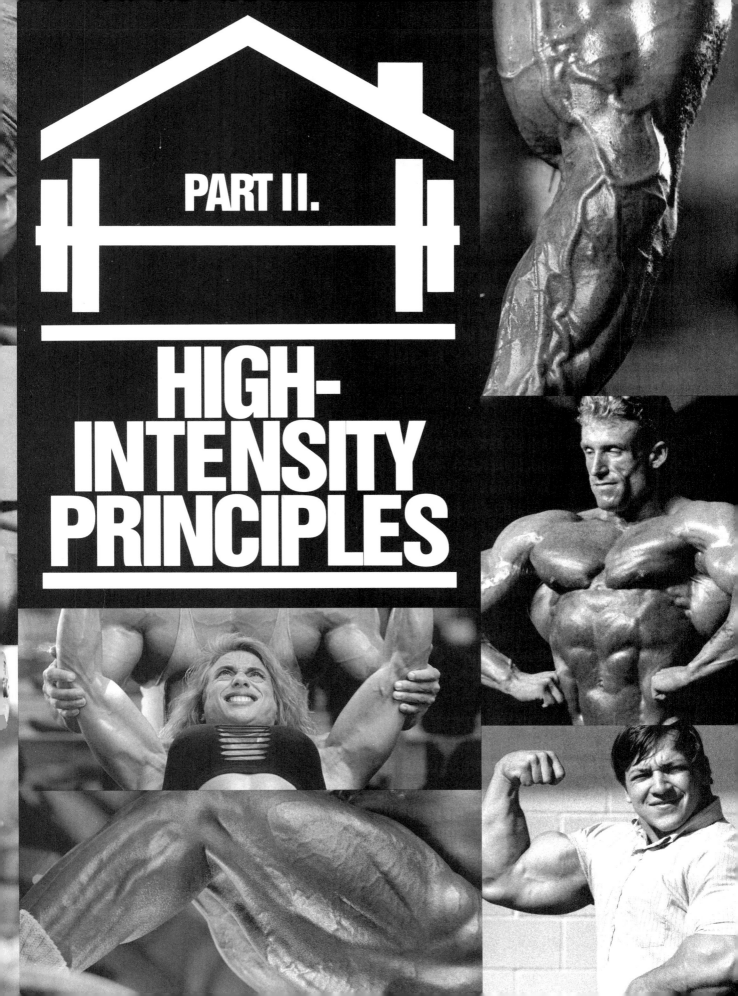

PART II.

HIGH-INTENSITY PRINCIPLES

CHAPTER 6
INTENSITY: ALWAYS HARDER

High-intensity exercise requires focused determination.

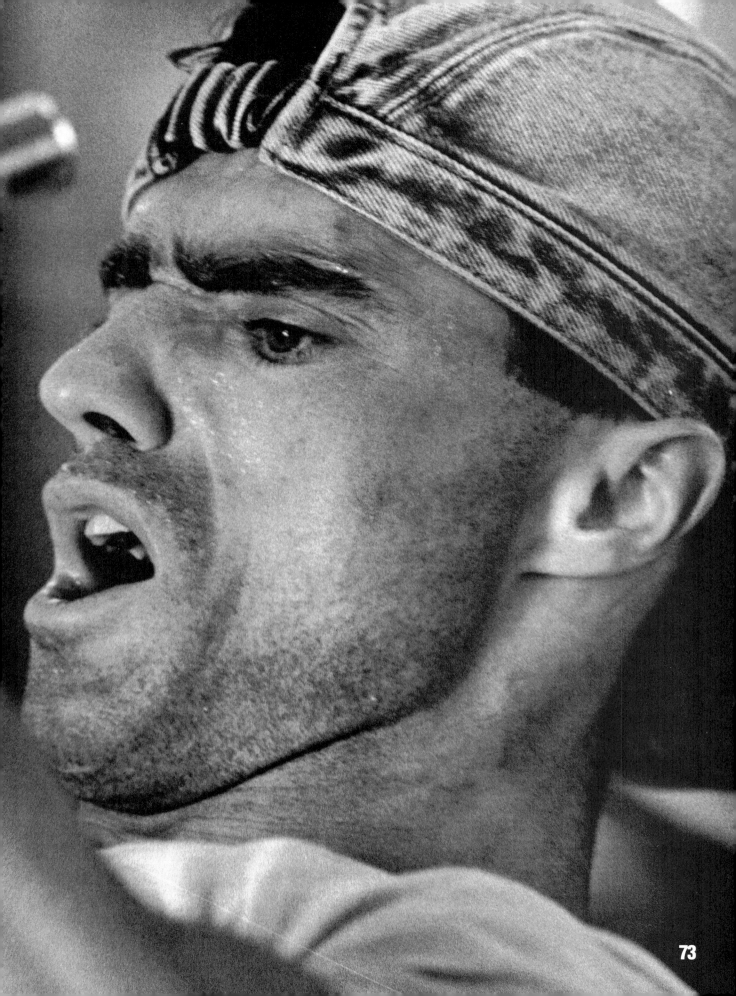

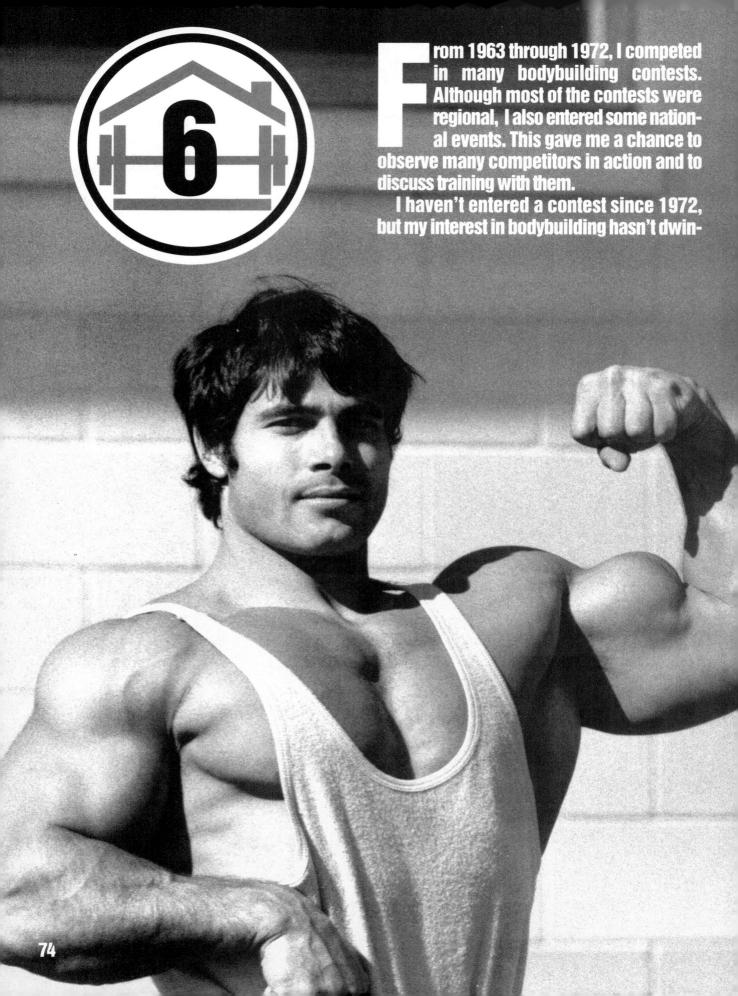

6

From 1963 through 1972, I competed in many bodybuilding contests. Although most of the contests were regional, I also entered some national events. This gave me a chance to observe many competitors in action and to discuss training with them.

I haven't entered a contest since 1972, but my interest in bodybuilding hasn't dwin-

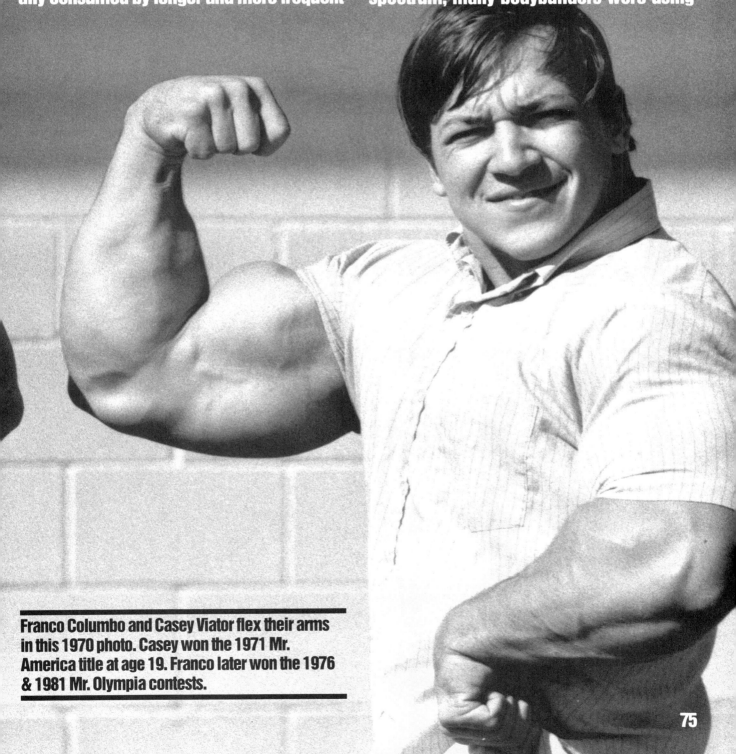

dled. I've continued to train, to travel, and to talk bodybuilding with interested people. Furthermore, I've done a lot of research and writing, and have published over two dozen books on the subject.

Over the last thirty years, I've seen a provocative trend emerge and disappear. During the 1960s, bodybuilders were gradually consumed by longer and more frequent training sessions, which were dubbed "marathon workouts." It got so extreme that one national-caliber athlete was spending eight hours a day training. He actually put up a tent in the gym so he could periodically prepare various foods and drinks and partake of them in privacy.

While this example is at the far end of the spectrum, many bodybuilders were using

Franco Columbo and Casey Viator flex their arms in this 1970 photo. Casey won the 1971 Mr. America title at age 19. Franco later won the 1976 & 1981 Mr. Olympia contests.

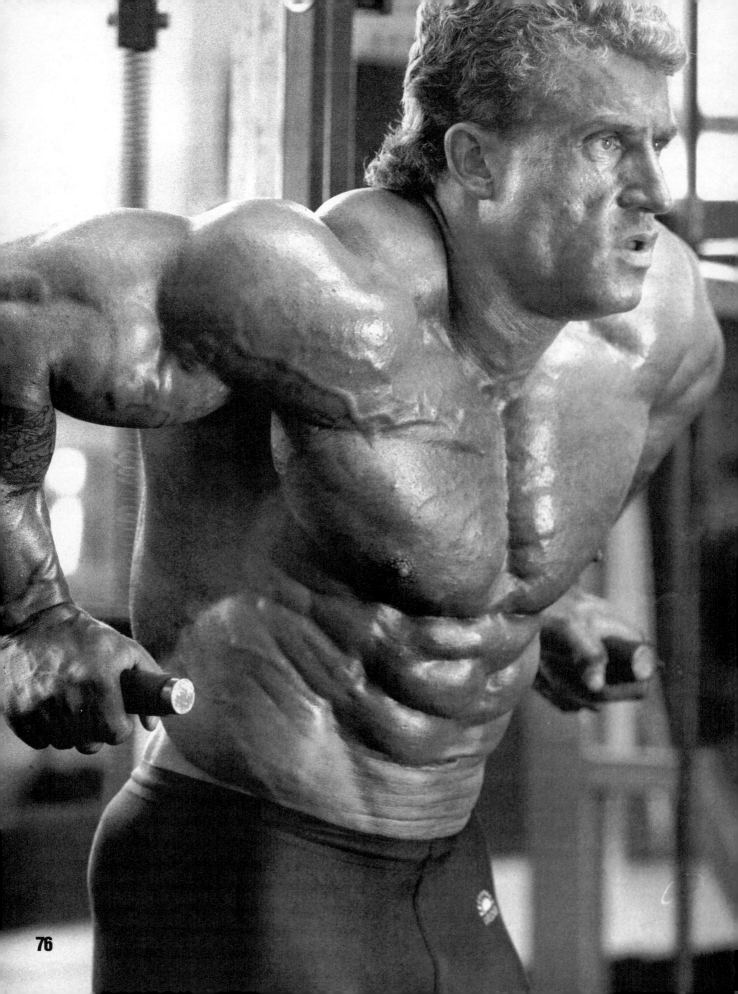

double-split routines, which required four hours per day to complete. These routines were repeated six days per week. Thus, their overall training time each week was twenty-four hours.

HARDER, BRIEFER TREND

In the 1970s, the marathon workout trend slowed and took a nosedive in the opposite direction. The primary cause of this nosedive were the writings of Arthur Jones. Jones's hard-hitting articles explained the advantages of harder, briefer, infrequent training. Jones advocated thirty-minute workouts, performed no more than three times per week. If that didn't produce immediate results, he reduced the workouts per week to only two. To prove his point, Jones personally trained Casey Viator on this radical philosophy for almost a year. In rapid succession, Viator won the 1970 Teenage Mr. America, 1970 Mr. USA, 1971 Jr. Mr. America, and—at age nineteen—1971 Mr. America. Casey Viator is the youngest winner ever of the Mr. America title.

It didn't take long for Arthur Jones and Casey Viator to have a large following. Jones's new company, Nautilus Sports/Medical Industries, reinforced the concepts by manufacturing machines that were physiologically correct for harder, briefer workouts.

Soon, hundreds of bodybuilders were applying Jones's guidelines to their training. Notable among this group were the Mentzer brothers, Mike and Ray. Both Mike and Ray went on to win Mr. America titles.

Dorian Yates of England is the new king of high-intensity training.

GENERAL FITNESS CROSSOVER

This harder-but-briefer philosophy steadily gained popularity over the next ten years, until it eventually crossed over into the general fitness market. Once fitness-minded men and women began to exercise in this fashion, it was only a short time before there were thousands of Nautilus Fitness Centers spread throughout the United States.

Around 1985 or so, the bodybuilding community again began moving toward longer, more frequent workouts. Today, as I visit gyms across the country, talk with trainees, and read the muscle magazines, I find that marathon workouts are back in style. Guys seem to be spending more and more time in the gym. The situation seems worse than ever.

THE EXCEPTION: DORIAN YATES

There is a notable exception to the marathon-workout craze. That's Dorian Yates, the 1992 winner of the Mr. Olympia.

In 1983, when Dorian first began bodybuilding, he was greatly influenced by Mike Mentzer's high-intensity training programs. Mentzer, a former Mr. America, had studied and practiced Arthur Jones's philosophy for many years.

Dedication to high-intensity training kept Yates's physique on a constantly upward path of development. In his first Mr. Olympia appearance, in 1991, he finished second to Lee Haney. Determined to win the title in 1992, Dorian traveled to California and worked out an entire month with Mentzer. Mike reinforced Dorian's doing only one all-out set per exercise. Consequently, Dorian's workouts for several months prior to the 1992 Mr. Olympia became harder and harder, and therefore briefer and briefer. I'm sure

Dorian's training time, compared to the other Mr. Olympia competitors, was much less. They probably exercised at least twice as much as he did.

If you look at the various photo coverages of the 1992 Mr. Olympia competition in Helsinki, you'll have to agree that Dorian Yates was the clear victor.

Dorian Yates, however, is an exception to the trend that has been sweeping the country for the last several years. Quantity, not quality; volume, not intensity—these seem to be the battle cries. For the rest of this chapter, I'll again focus on Arthur Jones.

OUTRIGHT HARD WORK

"Most bodybuilders don't know what hard work is," says Jones. "They're simply cowards. If you've never vomited from doing a set of curls, then you've never worked hard enough! There is only one way to maximum muscular size, and that one way involves outright hard work."

What is outright hard work in Arthur Jones's mind? I've observed Jones putting many bodybuilders through that one set of curls. Here's what usually happens:

- First, you select a weight on the barbell that you can perform for ten repetitions in good form. Jones would immediately decrease the weight by ten pounds just in case you overestimated your strength. Plus, it helped your confidence.

- Second, grasp the bar and stand erect. Anchor your elbows firmly against the sides of your waist and keep them there.

A front lat spread by Kevin Levrone, Shawn Ray, Dorian Yates, and Mohammad Benaziza.

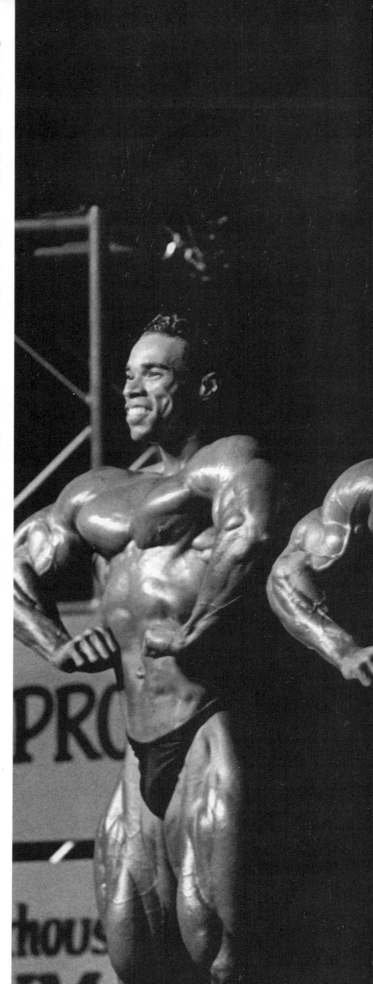

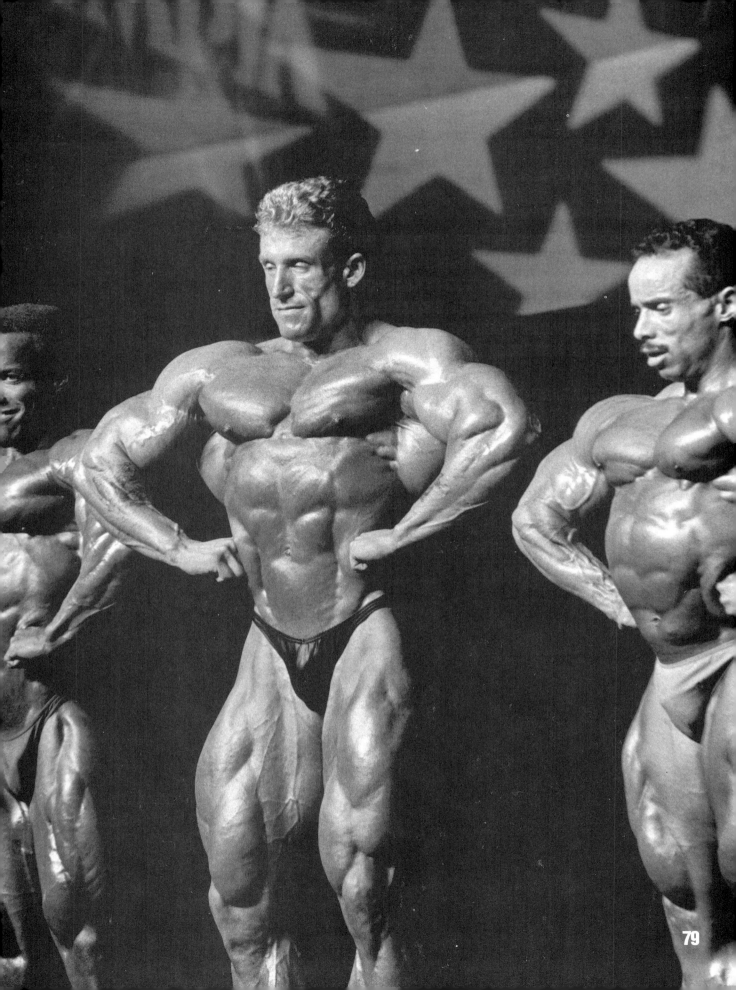

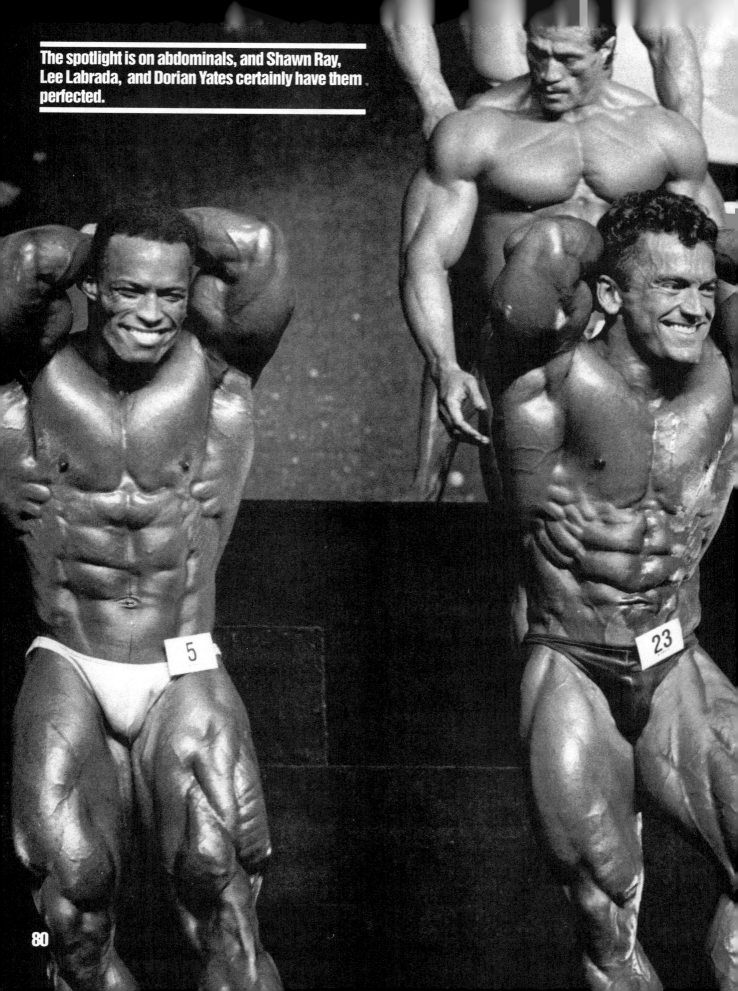

The spotlight is on abdominals, and Shawn Ray, Lee Labrada, and Dorian Yates certainly have them perfected.

5

23

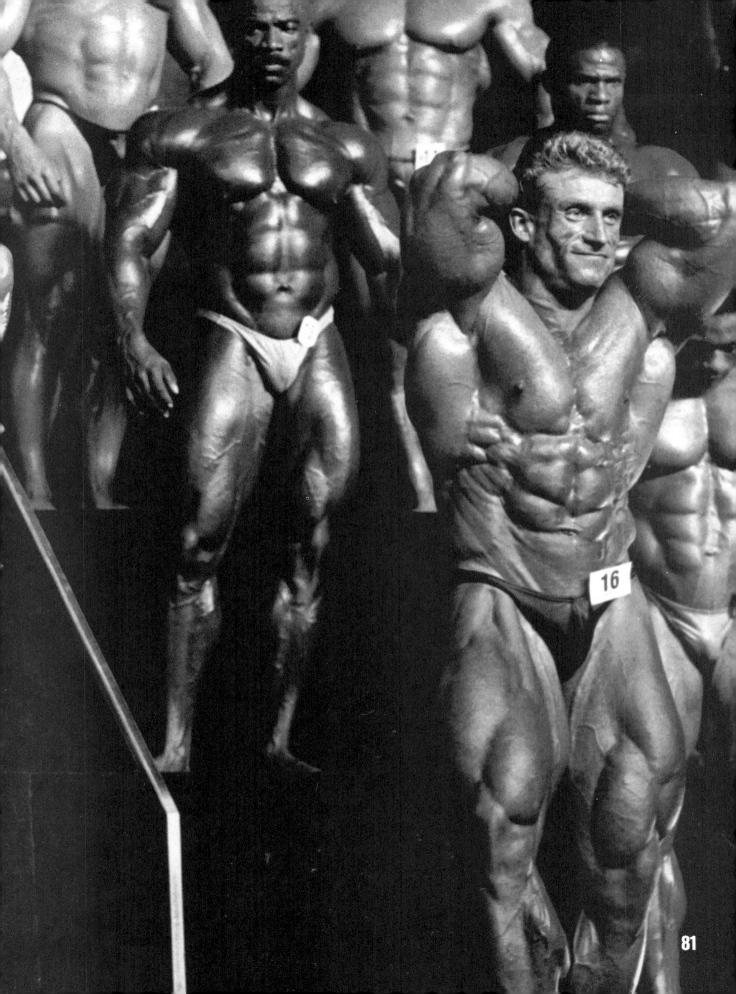

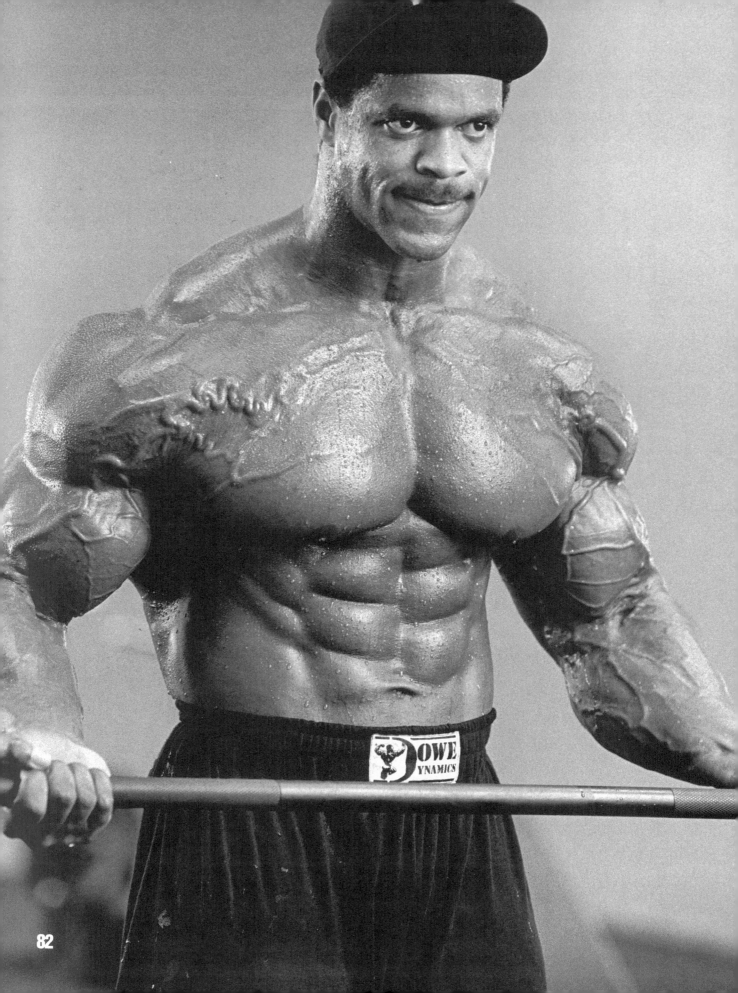

Lean forward slightly with your shoulders. Look down at your hands and curl the bar smoothly and slowly. Do not lean backward. Do not move your head. Pause briefly in the top position, but do not move your elbows forward. Keep your hands in front of your elbows. Lower the bar smoothly and slowly. Again, keep your elbows stable against your sides.

- Third, repeat the curling movements in the exact same form for ten repetitions. And since you selected the weight, you had better get ten repetitions—or you'll die. (Well, almost!)

- Fourth, no one ever gets ten repetitions in that form. No bodybuilder that I ever saw had ever done curls that strictly. You'll probably get about six reps and fail to complete the seventh. At that point Jones commands you, while you're still standing and holding the bar, to loosen your form slightly. Simply move your elbows a little. Sure enough, you can get another repetition that way. But now you fail to lift the eighth. By this point your biceps are very fatigued, and your forearms and hands are getting tired. Jones tells you to loosen your form more, to lean forward and backward a little while curling. Yep, you can do another, and with Jones insulting you, you get another. That was repetition eight and nine. Now your lower back is killing you, your legs are shaking, your lungs are burning, and your heart rate is over 200 beats per minute. Lucky for you, you've lost all feeling in your biceps, forearms, and hands.

Always look for little ways to make your exercise harder.

- Fifth, "just one more rep," as Jones says softly. He's even in front of you telling you he'll help you get that last repetition. Slowly the bar starts moving. You feel as if you're almost power-cleaning the barbell (which you are), with Jones assisting you (which he is). At the top, Jones gives a final command: "Bring the bar halfway down and hold for a count of five. That's it: five... four... three... two... one!"

In something less than one and a half minutes, you've experienced outright hard work from one set of ten repetitions of the barbell curl. And thirty minutes later, if you can get up off the floor, you'll still have a pump on your arms. And you'll feel much lighter without all that food in your stomach!

ALWAYS HARDER

Look for ways to make your exercise harder, not easier, and your overall results will always be better. This is one of the key components of high-intensity training.

Do not make the mistake of confusing intensity with the amount of exercise. A large amount of exercise cannot be high in intensity. Maximum-intensity exercise—just like the curling example described previously—because it is so exhausting, must be brief.

When an exercise is performed in a high-intensity manner, one set—and one set only—provides your body optimum stimulation. Multiple sets of the same exercise are not necessary.

Put 100 percent of your effort into that single set. Don't avoid the last repetitions in any exercise. Look forward to the increased intensity, endure the pain, and reap the results.

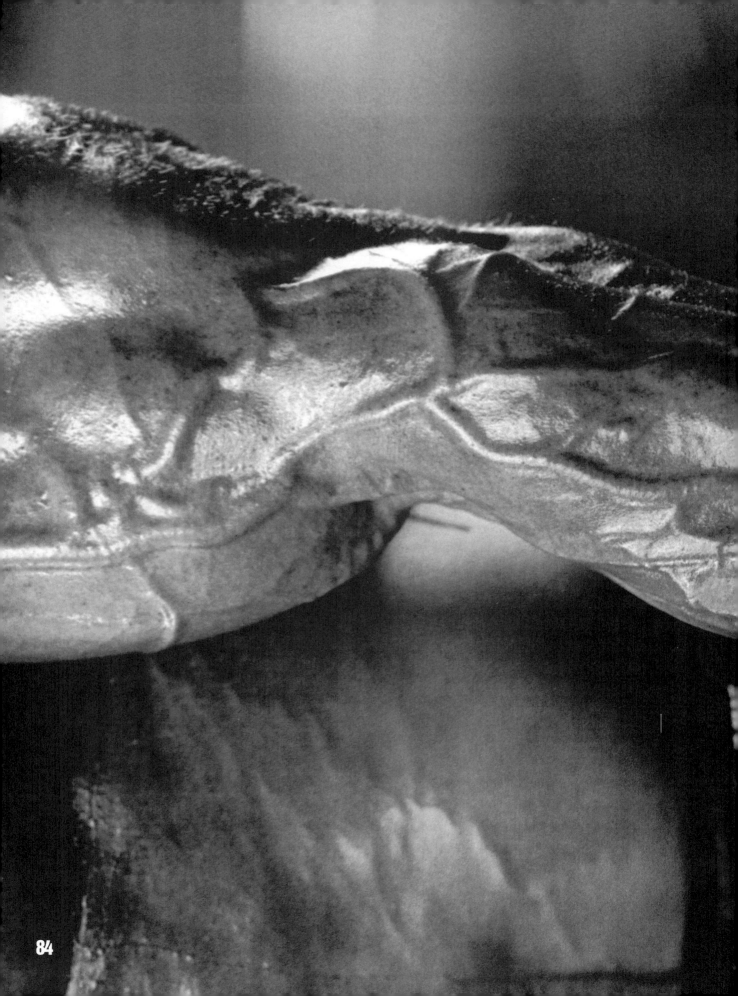

CHAPTER 7

PROGRESSION: POUND BY POUND

Strength equals size—and size equals strength. Your muscles must get stronger to get bigger.

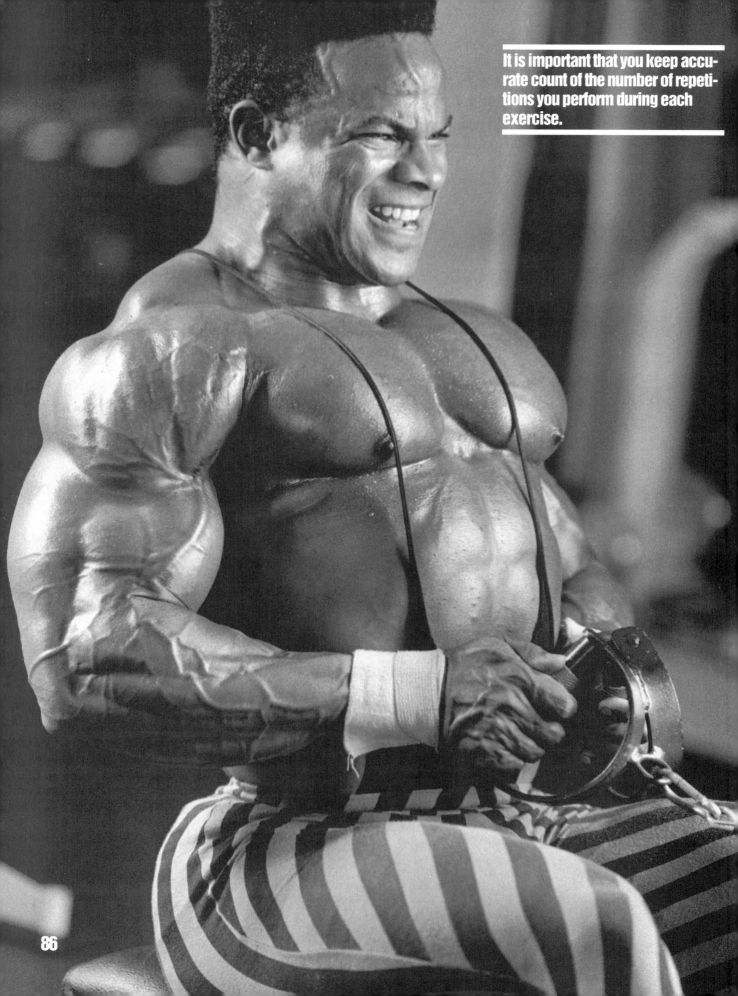

It is important that you keep accurate count of the number of repetitions you perform during each exercise.

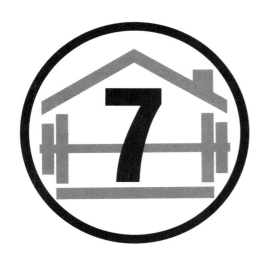

Visit any community in this country and organize a meeting of all the local bodybuilders. Then ask them to do two things. First, have each bodybuilder bring you his workout-by-workout training records for the last three months. Second, have each bodybuilder figure out the percentage of strength increase that he has made over the last three months on the basic exercises such as the bench press and the biceps curl.

You'll be amazed at what happens. The majority of bodybuilders in this country won't be able to produce training records of their workouts. The reason is they do not keep them—at least, not accurate training records.

Most of the bodybuilders who do have accurate training records will have a rate of strength increase per month of approximately 5 percent at best, and closer to 0 percent at worst.

In other words, most bodybuilders have poor training records and, as a result, it becomes very difficult to evaluate their progress. The bodybuilders that do keep training records are making little significant monthly progress in building strength.

STRENGTH EQUALS SIZE

Strength is important to a bodybuilder because it is the best way to determine progress. There is a direct relationship between muscular strength and muscular size. A stronger muscle is larger, and a larger muscle is stronger. Furthermore, it's easier to measure the strength of a muscle than its size.

The strength of a muscle is best measured, not by seeing how much you can lift one time maximally, but by determining how much you can lift ten times in good form. Thus, by comparing your ten-repetition sets for the same exercise to one another, you should be able to calculate your percent increase on a weekly and monthly basis.

5-PERCENT INCREASES

How much should your strength increase be on the bench press and biceps curl? Beginners should strive toward a 5-percent increase in each exercise per week, or approximately 20 percent per month. Advanced trainees should work toward a 5-percent increase in each exercise per two-week period, or approximately 10 percent per month.

Naturally, these increases will vary from exercise to exercise and from trainee to trainee, but the 5-percent increases per one-to-two-week time period are a reasonable goal. I've worked with hundreds of trainees who have reached these goals consistently for as long as three to six months before they reach a plateau.

PROGRESSIVE WEIGHT TRAINING

Progressive weight training—very simply, that's bodybuilding in a nutshell. But in

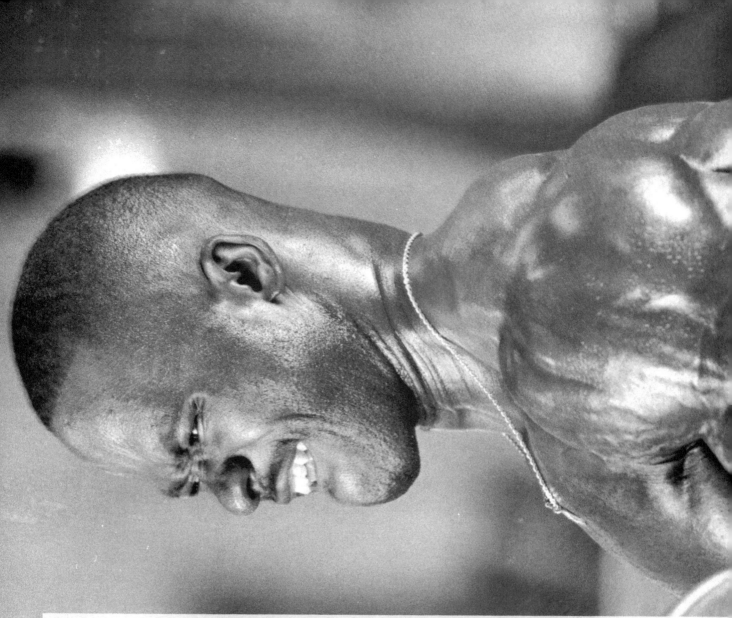

fact, there's little that is progressive about the training of most bodybuilders.

Don't let yourself get into the rut of performing the same number of repetitions with the same amount of weight workout after workout.

Be progressive.

Usually it is best to work between eight and twelve repetitions. Always try to do one or two repetitions more on each exercise today than you did in your last workout. When you can do twelve or more repetitions on an exercise, then increase the resistance by approximately 5 percent at your next training session. Small barbell plates that weigh 1 1/4 pounds and 2 1/2 pounds are important to have, especially at the beginning stage.

DOUBLE PROGRESSIVE TRAINING

This process is referred to as double progressive training, because first you add repetitions and then you add resistance.

Double progressive training is the backbone of all successful bodybuilding programs. As simple as the concept sounds, it's often ignored.

Understand and apply double progressive training in all your workouts and your results will be more significant. And remember,

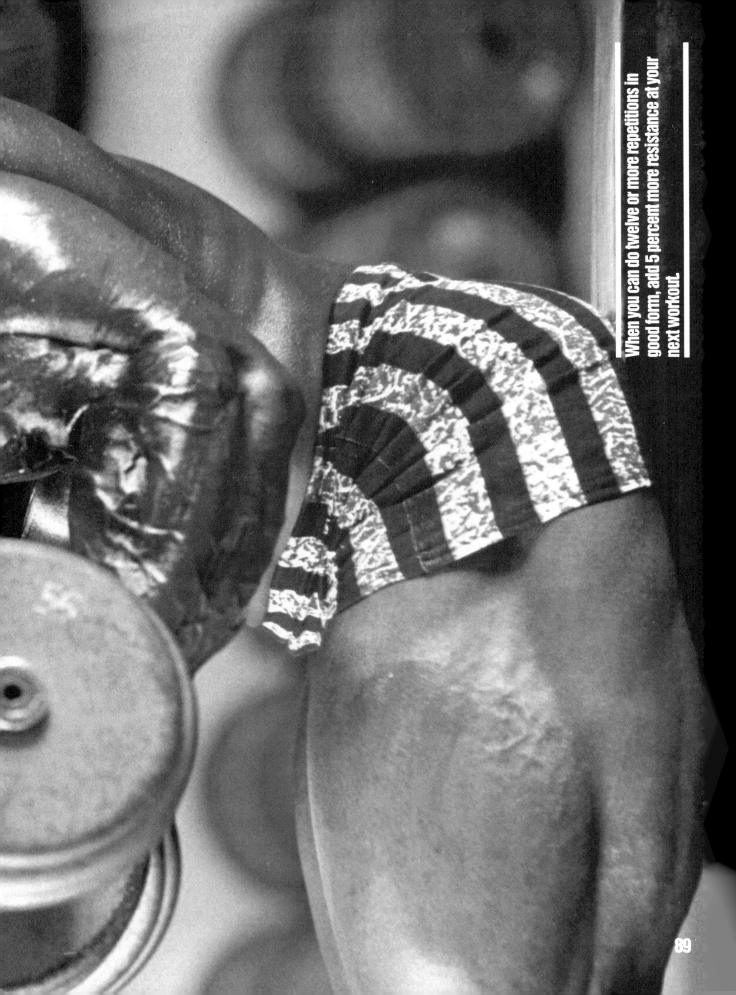

When you can do twelve or more repetitions in good form, add 5 percent more resistance at your next workout.

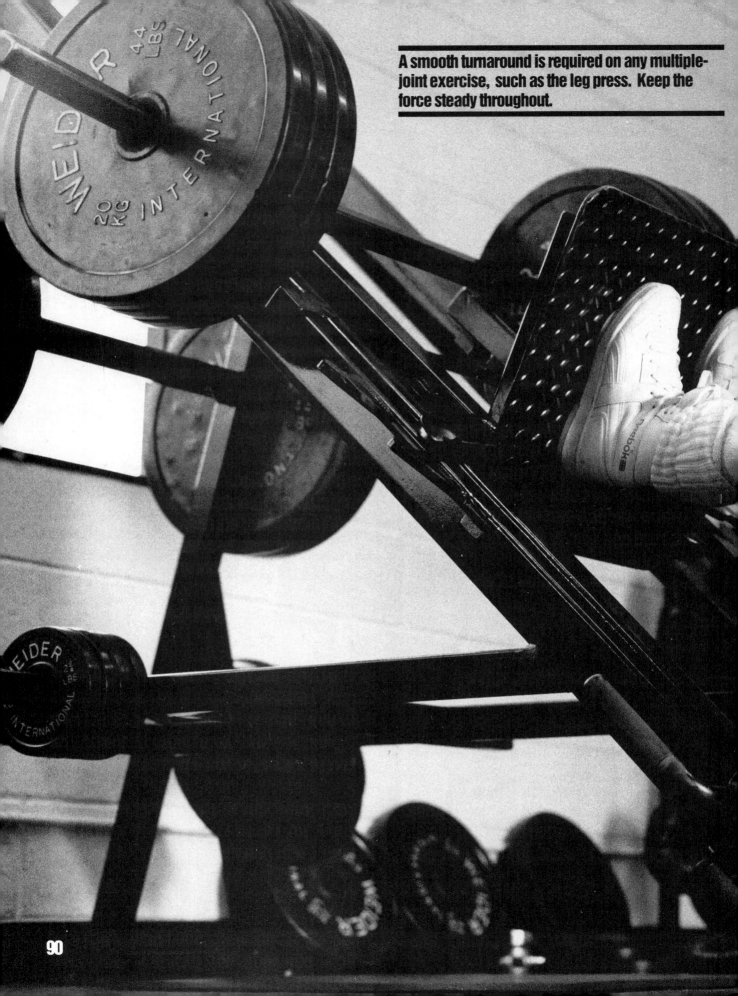

A smooth turnaround is required on any multiple-joint exercise, such as the leg press. Keep the force steady throughout.

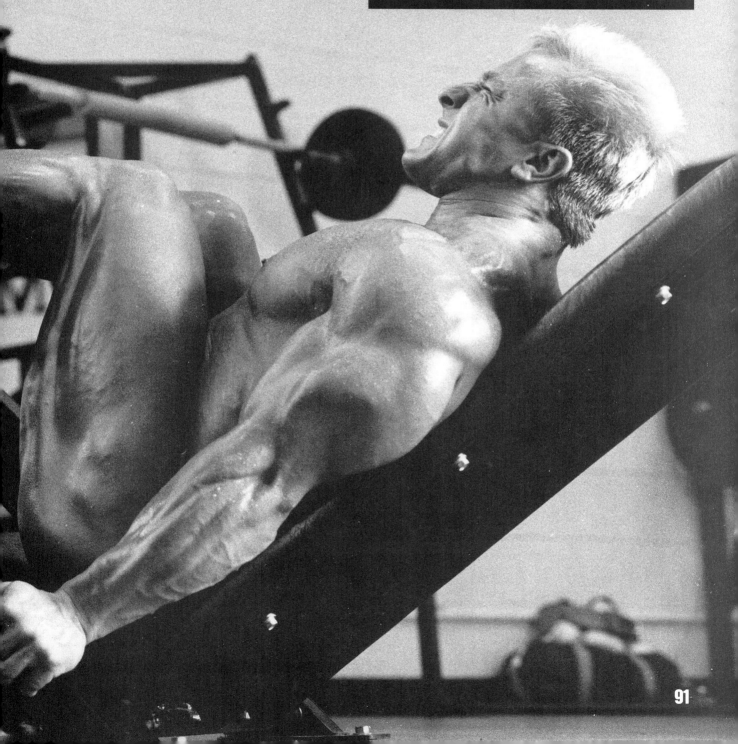

CHAPTER 8
FORM: SLOWER AND SMOOTHER

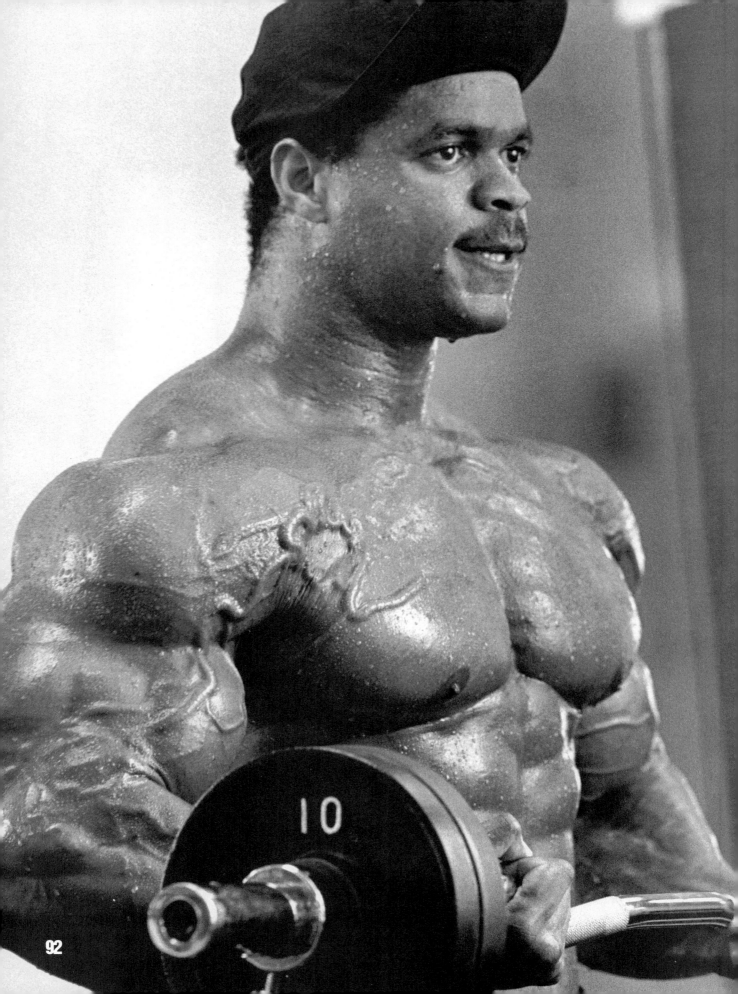

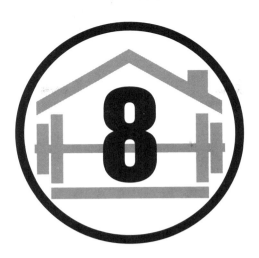

There is one thing that all bodybuilders everywhere do wrong—they perform repetitions too quickly. Correcting this one thing would produce better results instantly.

Slow down your speed of doing a repetition.

EXCESSIVE MOMENTUM

All bodybuilders lift the weight too quickly. They involve momentum at the start, which produces a forceful jolt on the muscle and joint. To stop the weight at the top, which is now partially out of control, requires more stress. Then the lowering phase of the repetition proceeds too fast and more transition force again occurs at the bottom as another repetition begins.

Three episodes of excessive force per repetition on the involved muscles, connective tissues, and joints—that's what happens hundreds of times per workout to every bodybuilder in the world. It's no wonder that so many bodybuilders get numerous aches and pains throughout their bodies as a result of their sloppy training.

Slow, smooth repetitions are not only safer, they are much more productive in stimulating your muscles to grow.

4 SECONDS UP, 4 SECONDS DOWN

What exactly do I mean by slow? I've experimented with various speeds of movement per repetition, such as 4 seconds, 6 seconds, 8 seconds, 15 seconds, 30 seconds, and even 60 seconds.

What works well with most barbell and free-weight exercises is 8 seconds per repetition. That's 4 seconds on the lifting or positive, and 4 seconds on the lowering or negative. There is a smooth turnaround at both the top and the bottom of the movement.

SLOW AND SMOOTH

The idea is to keep your targeted muscles overloaded throughout the entire set. Slow, smooth repetitions overload your muscles much better than faster styles, and they eliminate most of the momentum, which better isolates the involved muscles and makes the exercise harder.

Remember, the harder, stricter, and more targeted the exercise is, the better.

Although the weight you handle on any exercise is important, of equal importance is your style of lifting and lowering. When in doubt, always move slower.

CHAPTER 9
DURATION: LESS IS BETTER

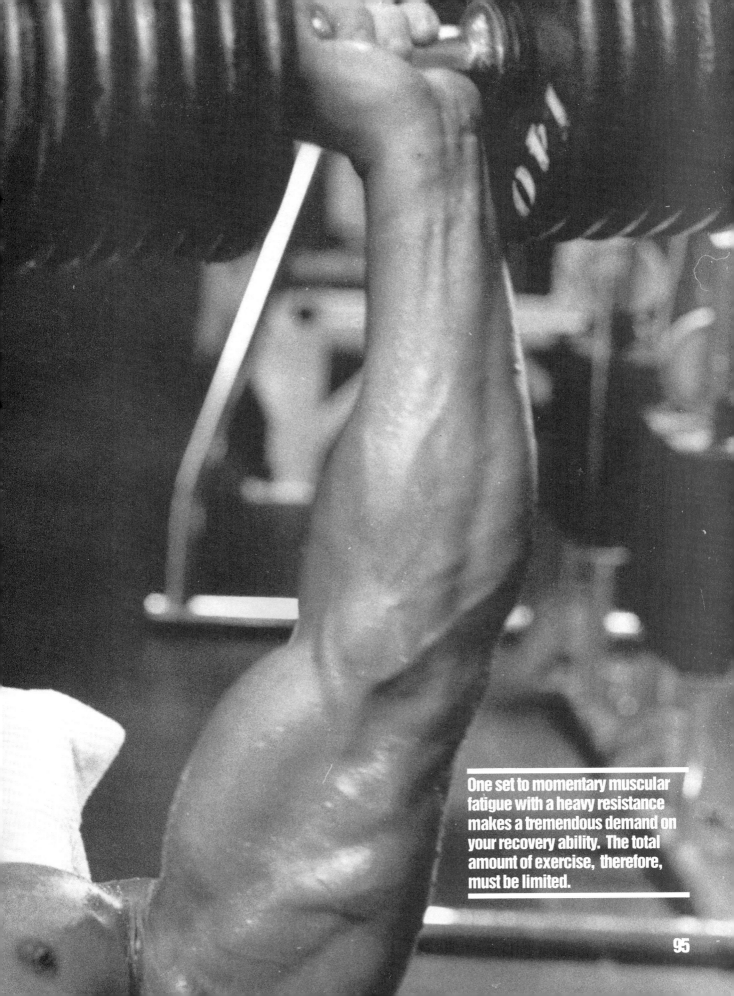

One set to momentary muscular fatigue with a heavy resistance makes a tremendous demand on your recovery ability. The total amount of exercise, therefore, must be limited.

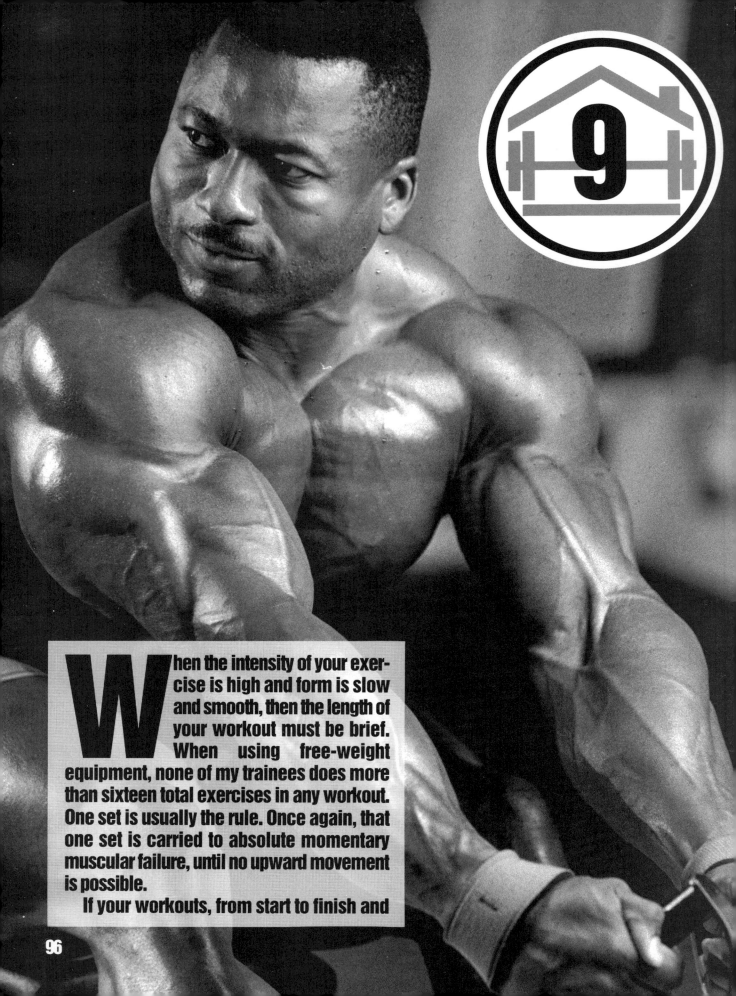

When the intensity of your exercise is high and form is slow and smooth, then the length of your workout must be brief. When using free-weight equipment, none of my trainees does more than sixteen total exercises in any workout. One set is usually the rule. Once again, that one set is carried to absolute momentary muscular failure, until no upward movement is possible.

If your workouts, from start to finish and

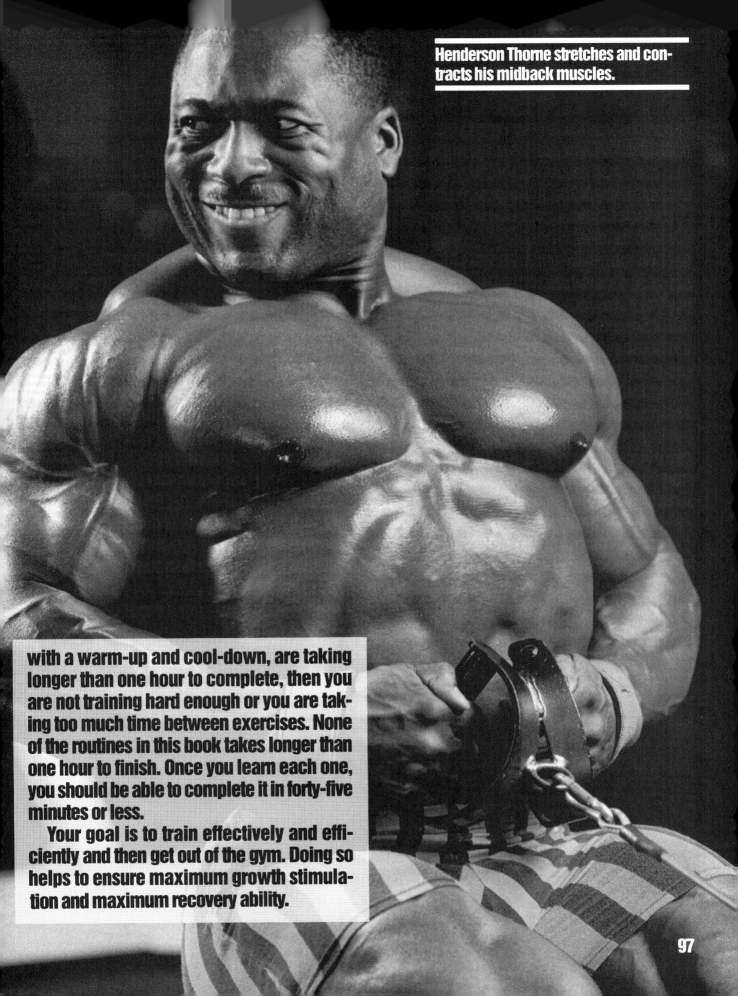

with a warm-up and cool-down, are taking longer than one hour to complete, then you are not training hard enough or you are taking too much time between exercises. None of the routines in this book takes longer than one hour to finish. Once you learn each one, you should be able to complete it in forty-five minutes or less.

Your goal is to train effectively and efficiently and then get out of the gym. Doing so helps to ensure maximum growth stimulation and maximum recovery ability.

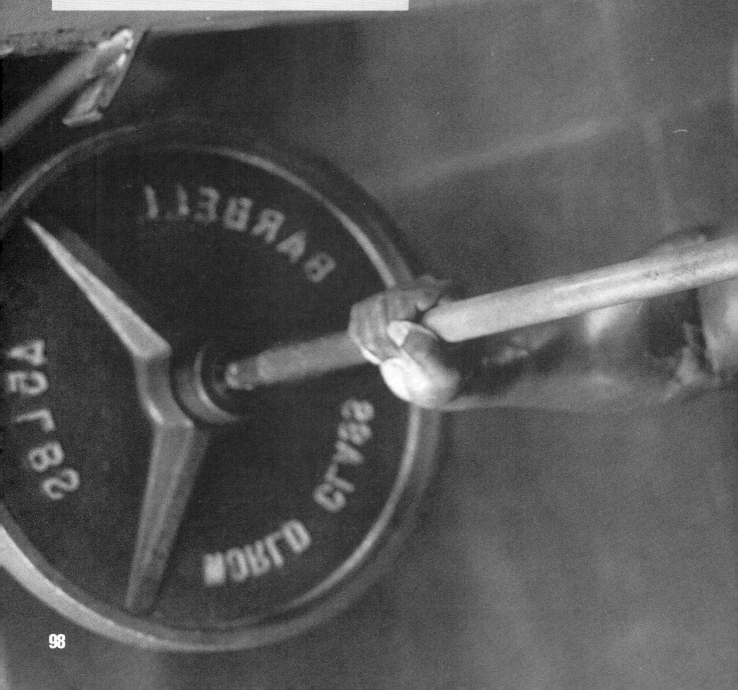

CHAPTER 10
FREQUENCY: THREE TIMES PER WEEK

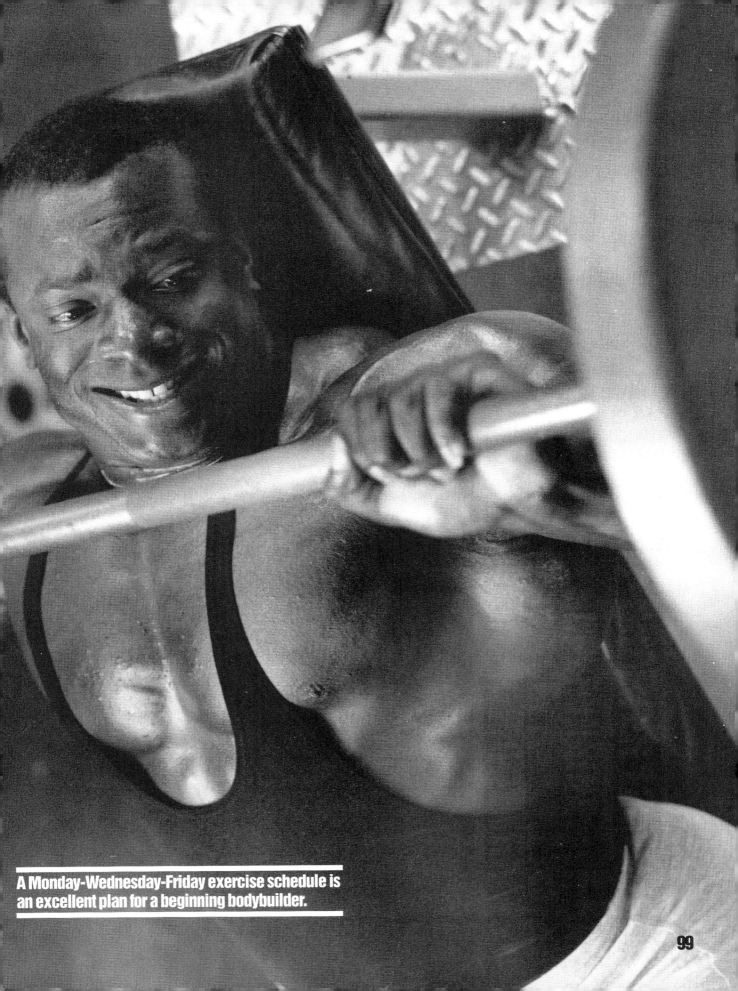

A Monday-Wednesday-Friday exercise schedule is an excellent plan for a beginning bodybuilder.

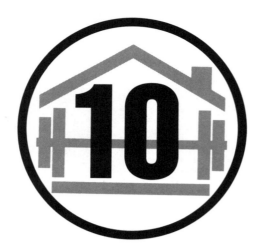

"Look at the muscular mass of a male lion," Arthur Jones said to me during a recent visit I had with him during the 1992 Christmas holidays. I had just asked if he had any new thoughts on optimum training frequency.

"A large male lion will weigh around five hundred pounds, while a large female will weigh only two hundred and fifty pounds," Jones continued. "And what kind of exercise schedule does each follow?"

"I didn't know lions exercised," I replied.

"Well, whether you call it work, or activity, or fighting, or chasing, or killing—they exercise. But there's a distinct difference between how the females exercise and how the males exercise.

"The females do the hunting. They stalk and kill game. Then they drag or carry the animals sometimes for miles to the dominant males. Of course, the females also take care of the young cubs when they're not hunting.

"The males, on the other hand, do only four things. They fight, mate, eat, and sleep. The males fight violently for territorial and mating rights. The fighting is very intense, but infrequent. And only the dominant male in each pride of lions mates with the females. The weaker males are killed or they leave the territory."

"In other words," I said, "what you're saying is one of the reasons that a male lion is twice the size of a female lion has to do with the male working harder, briefer, and more infrequently than the female."

"Yes," concluded Jones, "and the fact that the female daily does a large amount of continuous-type activity. She certainly doesn't rest and sleep nearly as much as does the male. The male probably sleeps fourteen hours a day."

Jones's discussion about lions convinced me more than ever that three workouts per week—three whole-body workouts, that is—are much more productive for bodybuilding than any type of split or double-split routine. Your stimulated body needs approximately forty-eight hours or more between workouts for consistent recovery overcompensation to occur. A Monday-Wednesday-Friday workout schedule is an excellent starting place. Such a schedule has proved effective over and over again.

"Tell your readers one last thing," Jones said as I was leaving. "Tell them that if three-times-per-week training doesn't produce the results they're after, they should work out only twice a week."

I thanked Arthur, opened the front door, and said good-bye to the female who was preparing the kill for Jones's evening meal.

Women should train with the same frequency as men.

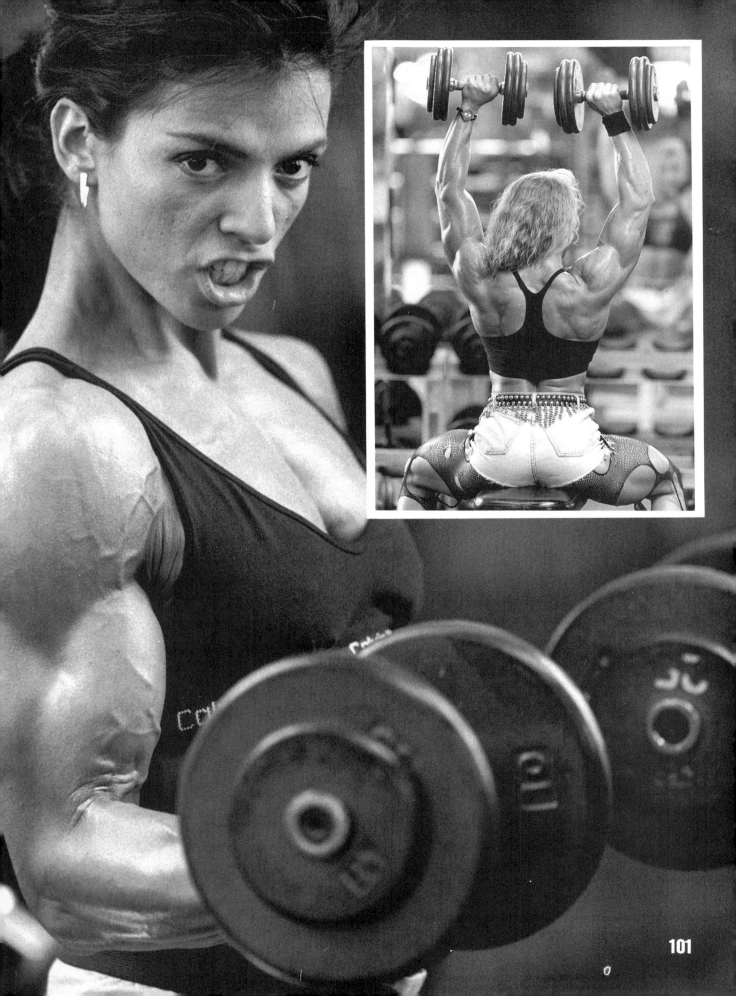

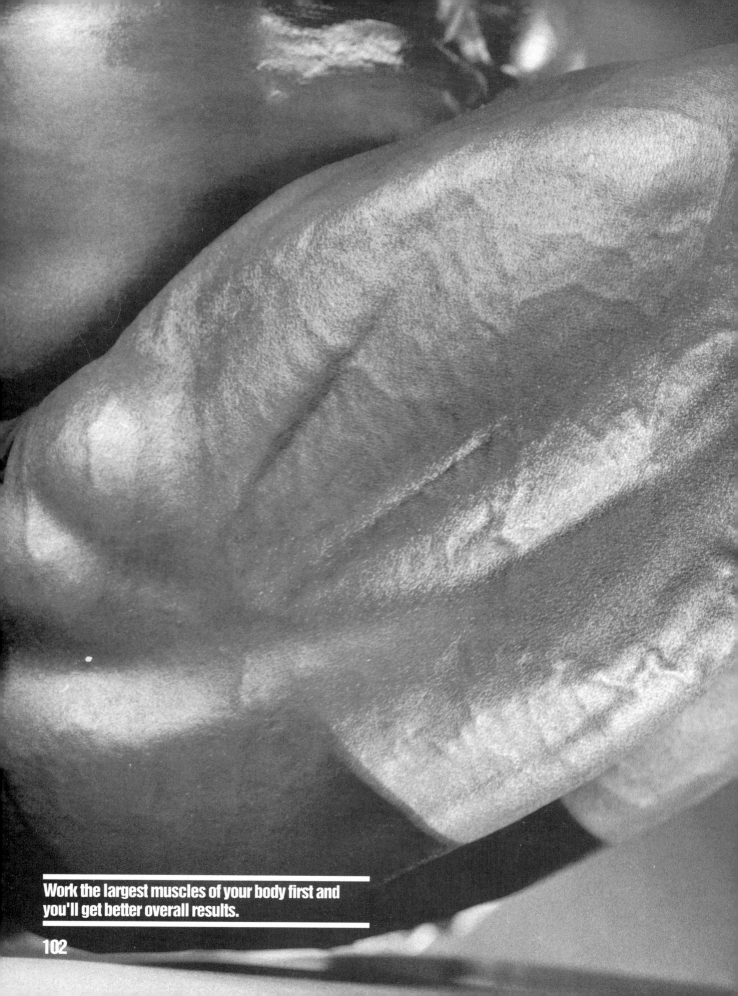

Work the largest muscles of your body first and you'll get better overall results.

CHAPTER 11
ORDER: LARGER TO SMALLER

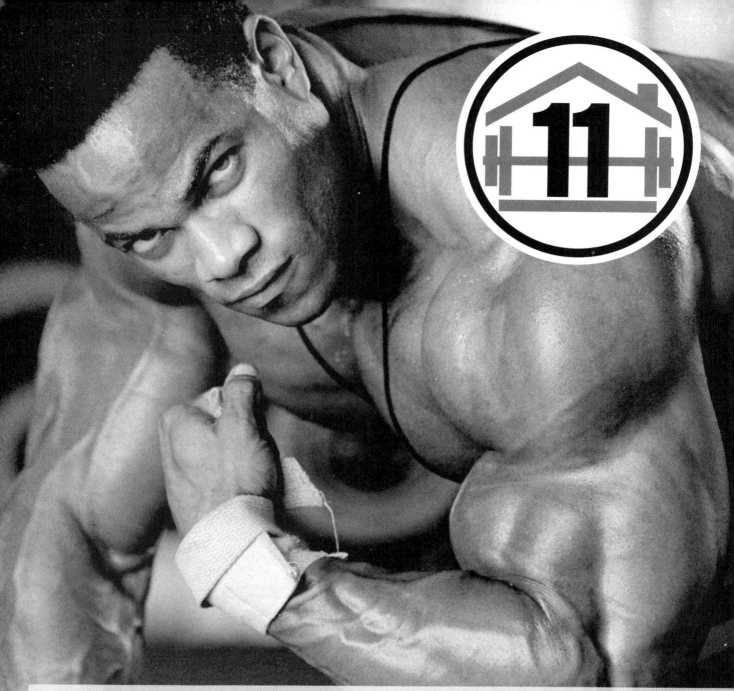

Many bodybuilders start their workouts with bench presses and curls, working the pecs and biceps, which are the show muscles in many trainees' minds. Toward the end of their workout, perhaps over an hour later, they might do a few leg exercises. Such a routine is a natural mistake, but a mistake nonetheless.

The average bodybuilder isn't going to build much muscle mass on his pectorals and biceps unless first considerable amounts of muscle have been developed around his hips, thighs, and back. It isn't possible to add significant muscular size in the small body parts unless the big body parts are growing as well. In fact, your smaller body parts often progress in proportion to the increase in size of your larger body parts,

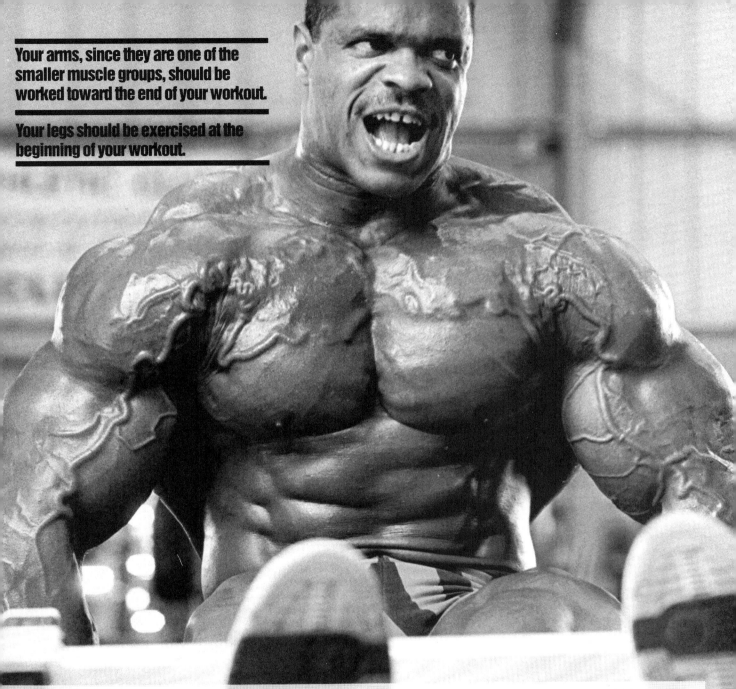

Your arms, since they are one of the smaller muscle groups, should be worked toward the end of your workout.

Your legs should be exercised at the beginning of your workout.

even if you don't work the small areas.

Thus, for many months, a bodybuilder's greatest concentration should be directed toward working his largest muscles first, when he should be strongest and most motivated. If his enthusiasm runs low and he has to neglect something, he's usually better off skipping his smallest muscle groups, which he normally saves until the end of his routine.

The ideal order of exercise is to work your lower body before your upper body, your hips and thighs before your calves, your back before your chest, and your upper arms before your forearms. Since your waist muscles stabilize your upper body in most exercises, work them last.

There are a few exceptions to the larger-to-smaller guideline, and they will be addressed in Part V, where specialized routines are discussed.

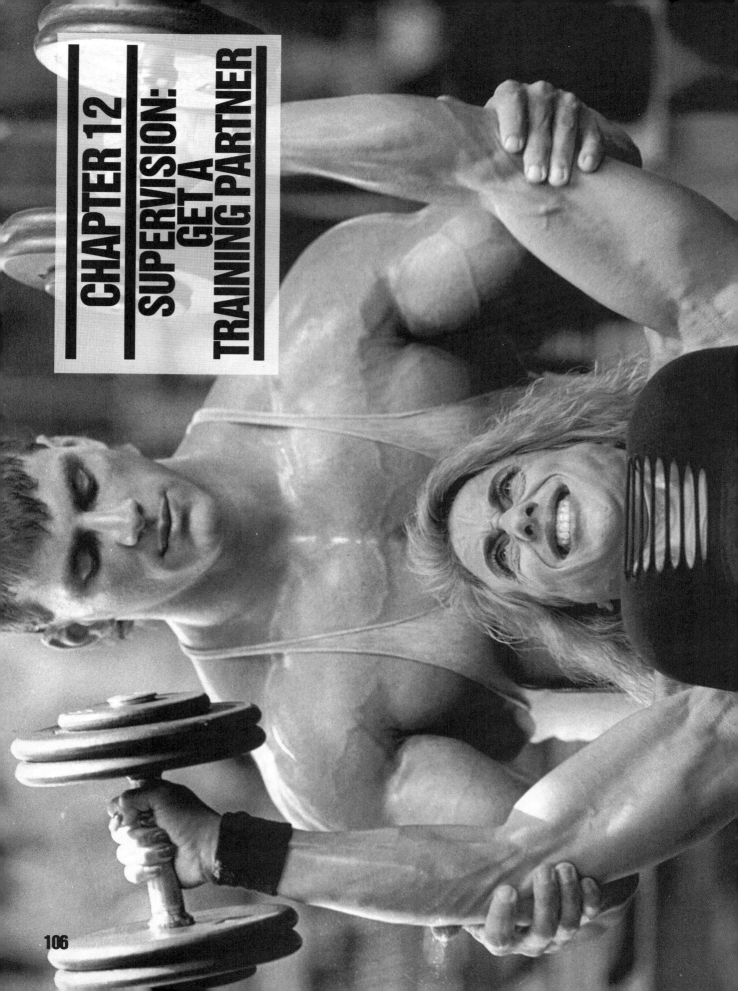

CHAPTER 12
SUPERVISION: GET A TRAINING PARTNER

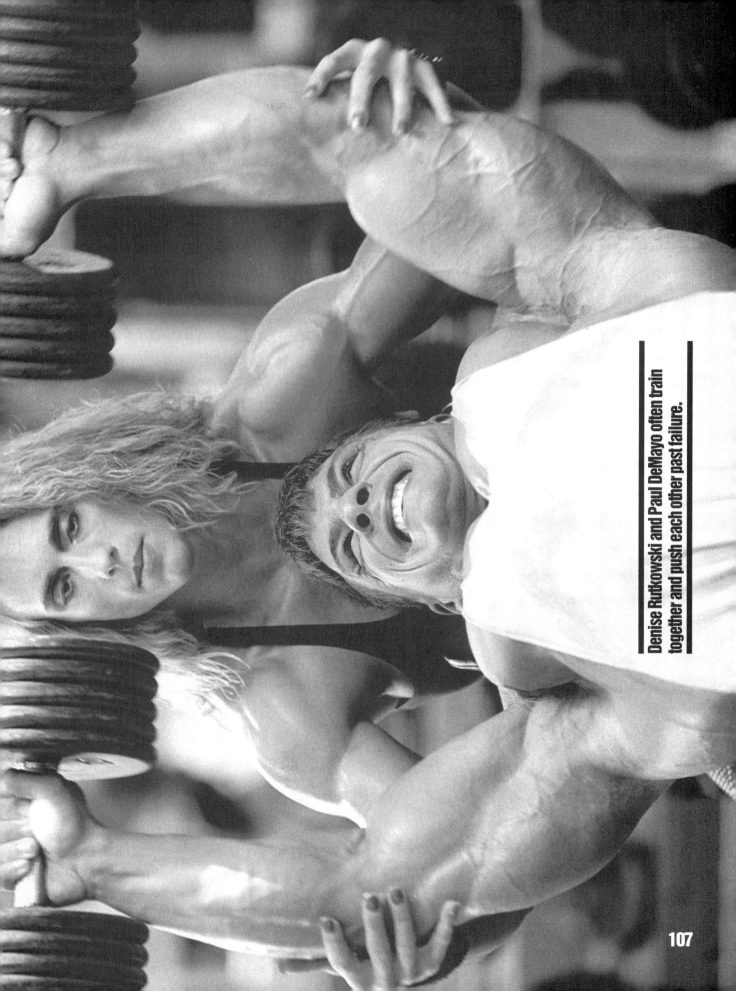

Denise Rutkowski and Paul DeMayo often train together and push each other past failure.

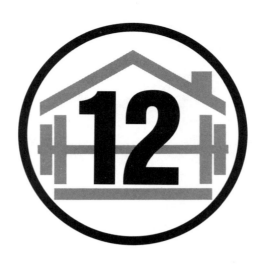

In my more than thirty years of training, I've observed only two men who could push themselves consistently to an all-out effort. One was Dick Butkus, the all-pro middle linebacker for the Chicago Bears. The other was Dan Gable, the world and Olympic-champion freestyle wrestler from the University of Iowa. Their training savvy was one of the main reasons they were superstars in their specific sports.

Very few bodybuilders push themselves to the limit, especially in the most demanding exercises, such as the squat and deadlift. Sure, you can probably push yourself to failure in two or three of the easier-to-do exercises in a selected workout. But to do it in every exercise in every workout for a month? That's almost impossible.

It takes a supervisor to push, urge, implore, and even bully you to do every repetition—and then one more—as well as to help you adhere to the strictest style possible. Most of you will never have your own private coach, but you can work with the next best thing: a training partner.

Bodybuilding with a serious partner will make a significant difference in your overall results. This person should be dedicated to ensuring that you get the most out of all your routines. While it's not imperative that you're of similar strength, if you are training on very similar routines, it's preferred.

Whatever pain your training partner inflicts upon you, give it back when it's your turn to supervise. With some good training charts and recordkeeping, both of you should soon know what high-intensity training is about.

After both of you have trained, one person going through the entire workout and then the other doing the same, sit down and briefly evaluate the workouts. Did you really go all-out on the chin-up? Wasn't there another rep in you? What about the stiff-legged deadlift? Couldn't you have tolerated the pain for another couple of repetitions? As you can see, I'm talking about full-bore training—the kind that produces enormous results, quickly!

While it's possible to make gains without a training partner, a motivated and serious person can make a great difference. Do what you can to find such an individual.

Porter Cottrell is ready to assist Steve Brisbois as he does a set of close-grip pulldowns.

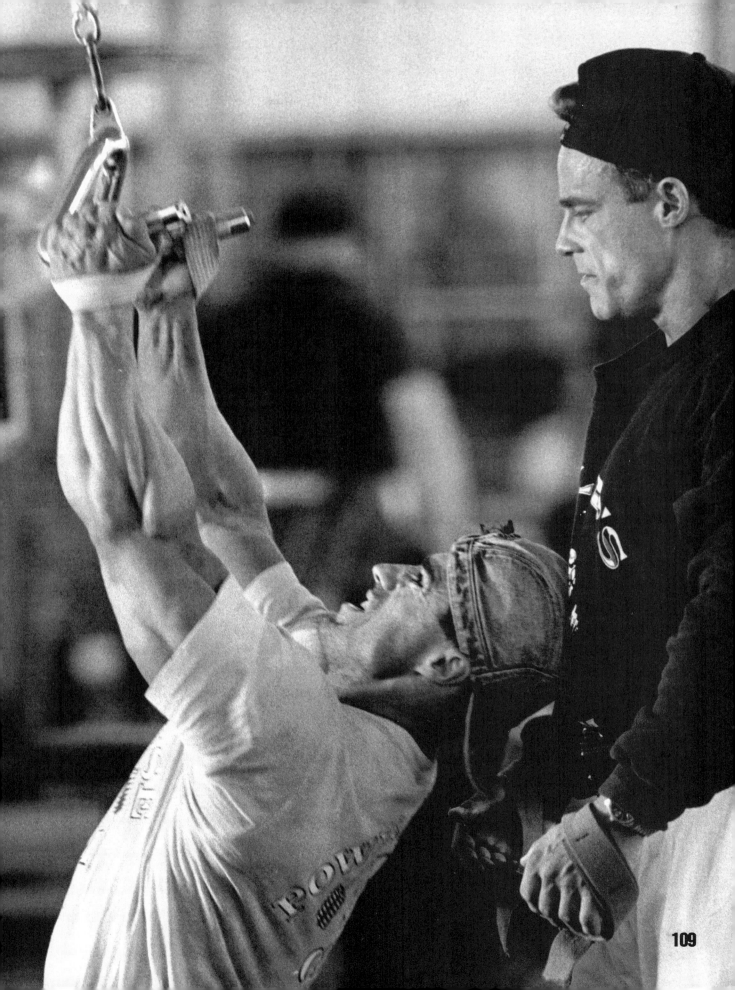

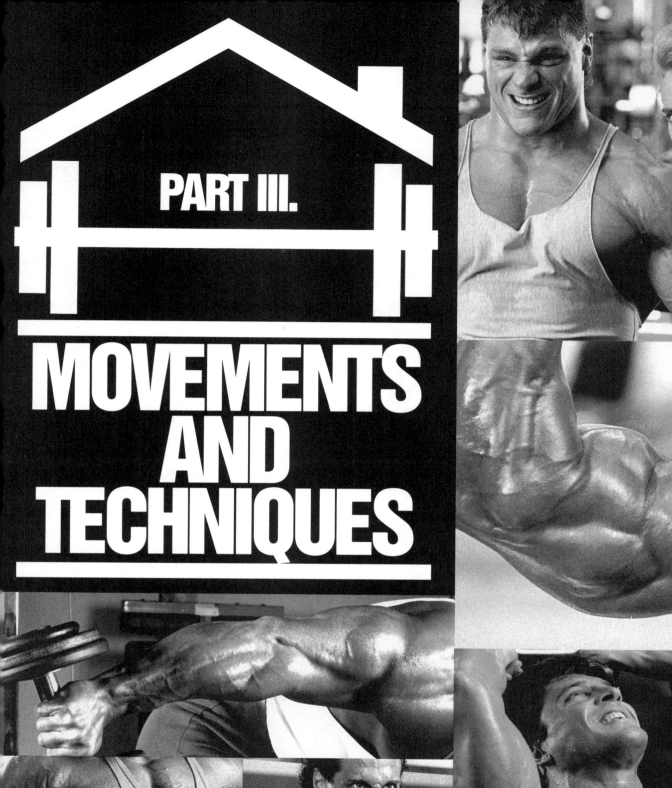

PART III.

MOVEMENTS AND TECHNIQUES

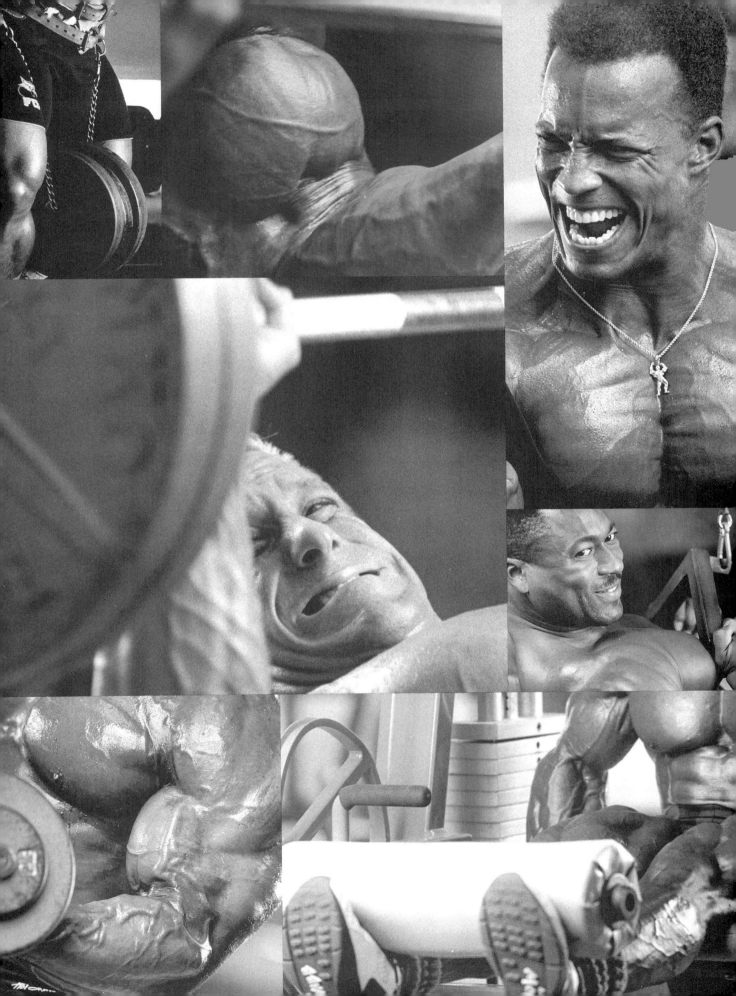

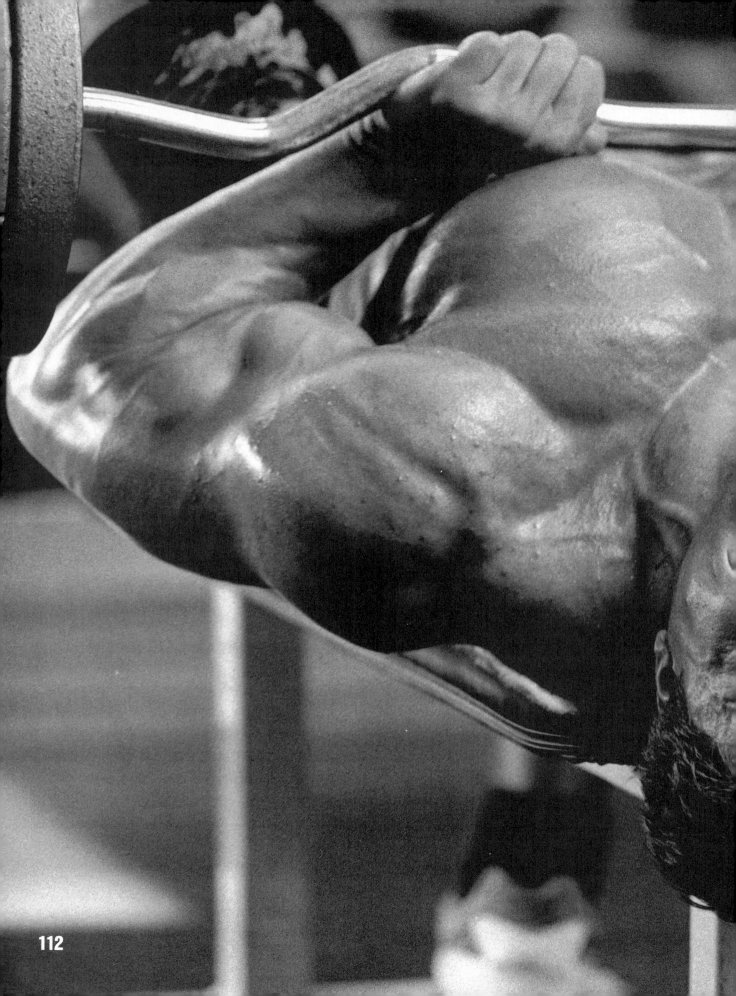

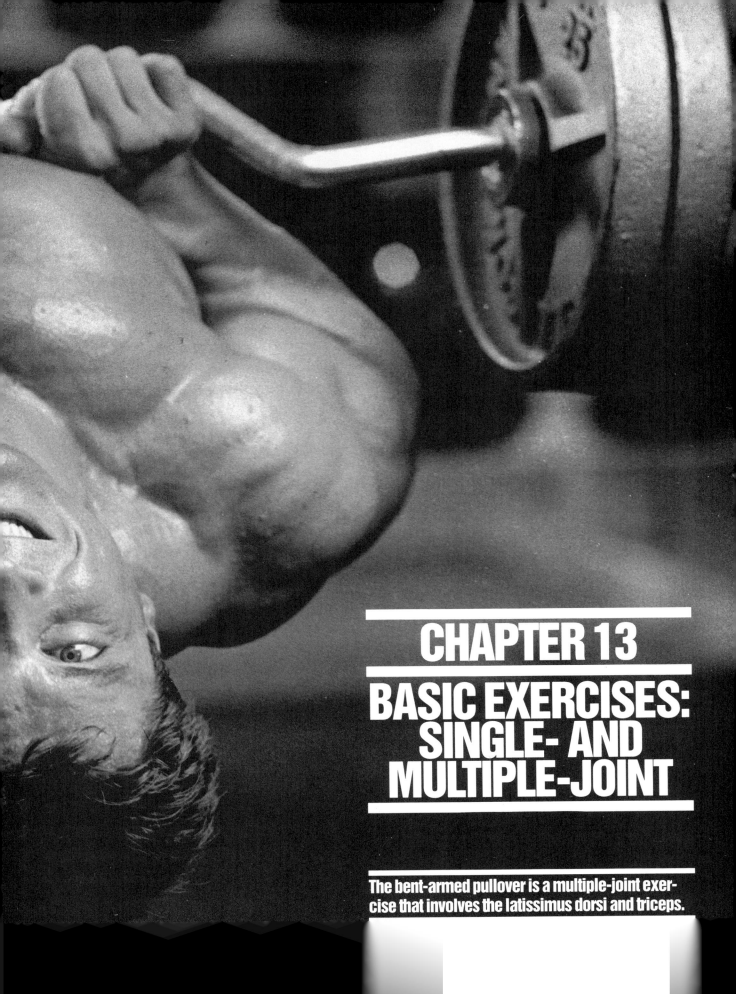

CHAPTER 13
BASIC EXERCISES: SINGLE- AND MULTIPLE-JOINT

The bent-armed pullover is a multiple-joint exercise that involves the latissimus dorsi and triceps.

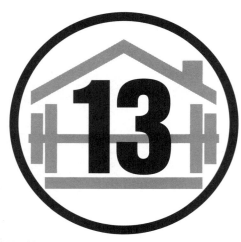

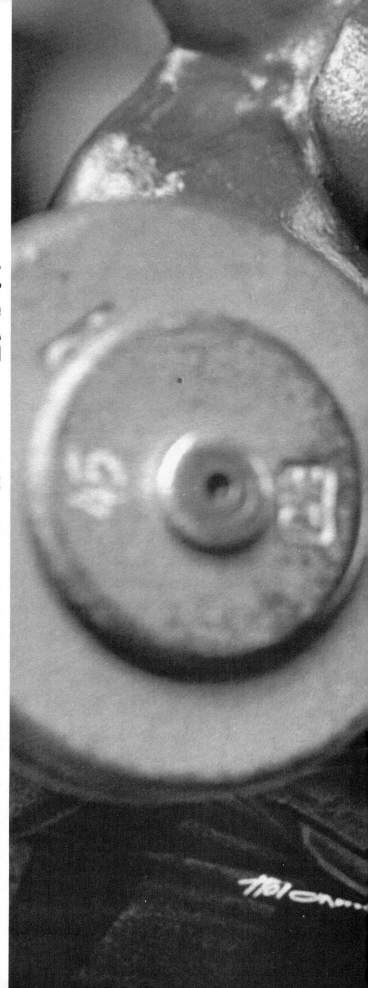

There are dozens and dozens of exercises that you can perform in your home gym. Some, however, are much more productive than others. A few, because of their danger, should be avoided.

SINGLE- AND MULTIPLE-JOINT MOVEMENTS

The basic bodybuilding exercises can be grouped under two headings: single-joint movements and multiple-joint movements. Single-joint movements involve only one joint. A triceps extension, with rotation around the elbows, is an example of a one-joint exercise. Multiple-joint movements require work around two or more joints. The bench press, for example, stresses the wrists, elbows, and shoulders.

Both single-joint and multiple-joint exercises are important to your bodybuilding program. You should understand, however, that each has a different effect on the involved muscles.

A single-joint exercise does a much better job of isolating a targeted muscle, such as the triceps. Strict performance of the triceps extension, with no elbow sway, will produce a thorough congestion in the backs of your upper arms.

A multiple-joint exercise involves some

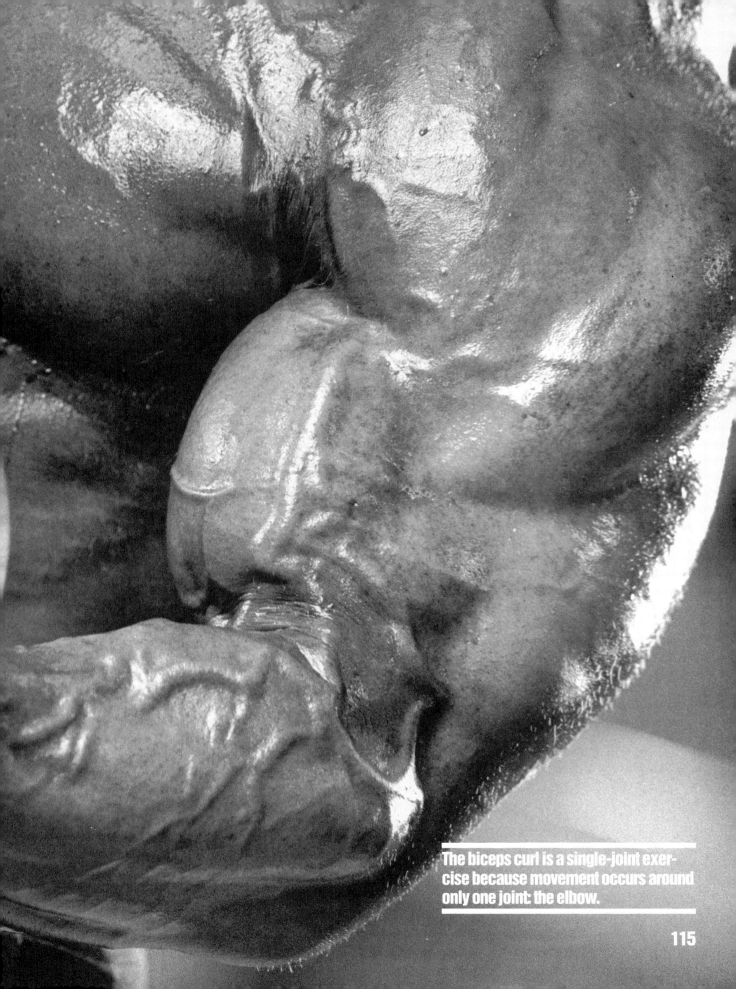

The biceps curl is a single-joint exercise because movement occurs around only one joint: the elbow.

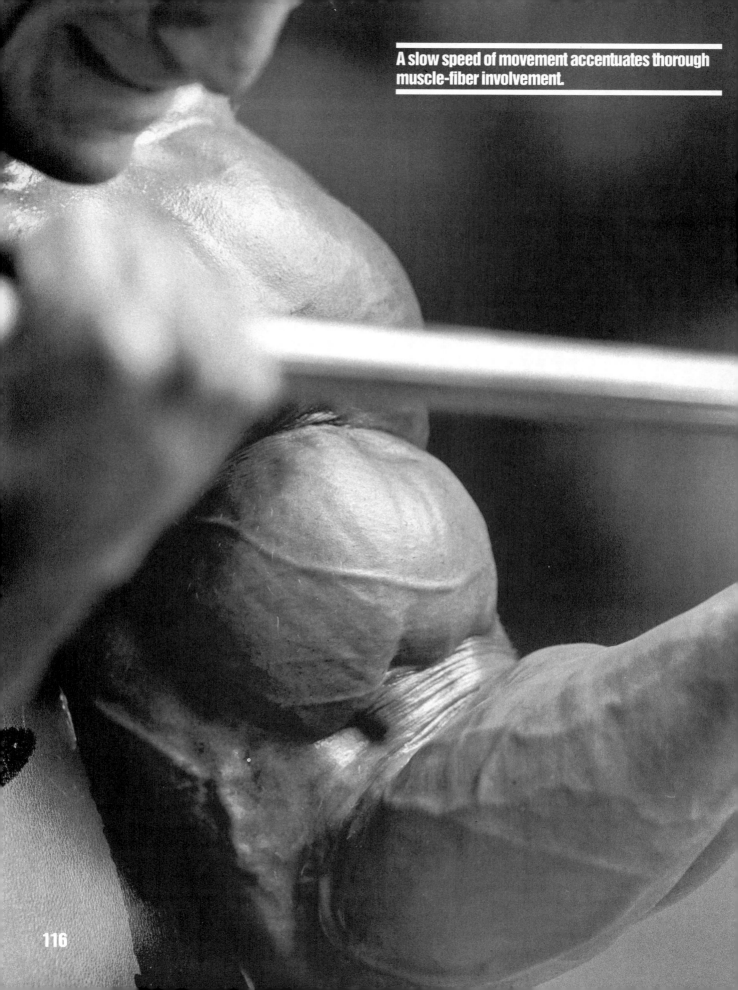

A slow speed of movement accentuates thorough muscle-fiber involvement.

work for many muscles, but it does not work any one muscle group thoroughly. The bench press stresses your triceps, front deltoids, and pectorals in a limited, midrange fashion. It doesn't involve any of these muscles throughout as long a range of movement as does a more specific single-joint exercise, such as the triceps extension for the triceps, the front raise with dumbbells for the anterior deltoids, and the straight-armed fly with dumbbells for the pectorals.

The benefit of the bench press, and other multiple-joint exercises, is that it brings into action more total muscle mass. You can use a much heavier resistance on a multiple-joint movement than on a single-joint movement. Thus, the overall growth effect on your body is greater.

Obviously, for best growth stimulation, your body requires both types of exercise. Let's examine the best single-joint and multiple-joint movements.

BEST EXERCISES

The best home-gym exercises, and the muscles worked in each, are listed below. They should be primary in most of your bodybuilding routines. The majority of these exercises are described fully in later chapters.

SINGLE-JOINT MOVEMENTS

- Calf raise (gastroc-soleus)
- Donkey calf raise (gastroc-soleus)
- Trunk curl (rectus abdominis)
- Reverse trunk curl (rectus abdominis)
- Shoulder shrug (trapezius)
- Lateral raise (middle deltoids)
- Front raise (front deltoids) ANTERIOR
- Bent-over raise (back deltoids)
- Straight-armed pullover (latissimus dorsi)
- Straight-armed fly (pectoralis majors)
- Biceps curl (biceps)

- Reverse curl (brachialis, biceps, and forearm extensors)
- Triceps extension (triceps)
- Bent-over triceps kickback (triceps)
- Wrist curl (forearm flexors)
- Reverse wrist curl (forearm extensors)

MULTIPLE-JOINT MOVEMENTS

- Squat (gluteals, quadriceps, hamstrings, and erector spinae)
- Hack squat (gluteals, quadriceps, and hamstrings)
- Sissy squat (quadriceps)
- Stiff-legged deadlift (hamstrings, gluteals, and erector spinae)
- Deadlift (hamstrings, gluteals, and erector spinae)
- Chin-up (biceps and latissimus dorsi)
- Behind-neck chin-up (biceps and latissimus dorsi)
- Dip (triceps, deltoids, and pectoralis majors)
- Overhead press (triceps and deltoids)
- Press behind neck (triceps and deltoids)
- Upright row (deltoids and trapezius)
- Bent-over row (biceps and latissimus dorsi)
- Bench press (triceps, deltoids, and pectoralis majors)
- Decline press (triceps, deltoids, and pectoralis majors)
- Incline press (triceps, deltoids, and pectoralis majors)
- Bent-armed fly (pectoralis majors and triceps)
- Bent-armed pullover (triceps and latissimus dorsi)

Naturally, there are variations of many of these basic exercises. The most effective variations are recommended in later chapters.

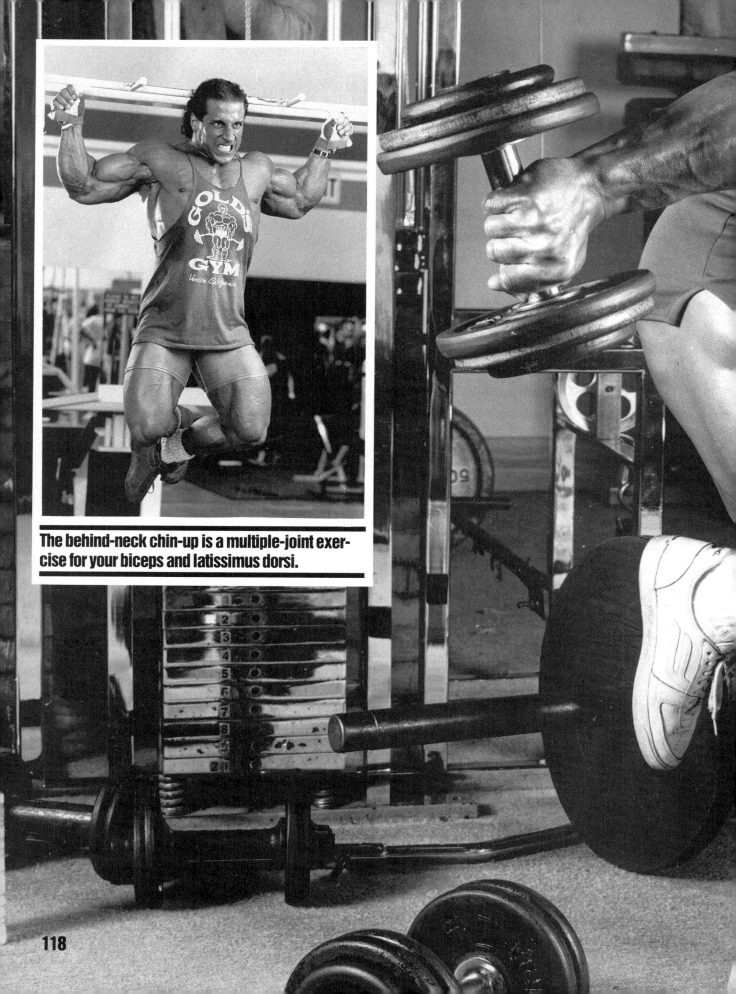

The behind-neck chin-up is a multiple-joint exercise for your biceps and latissimus dorsi.

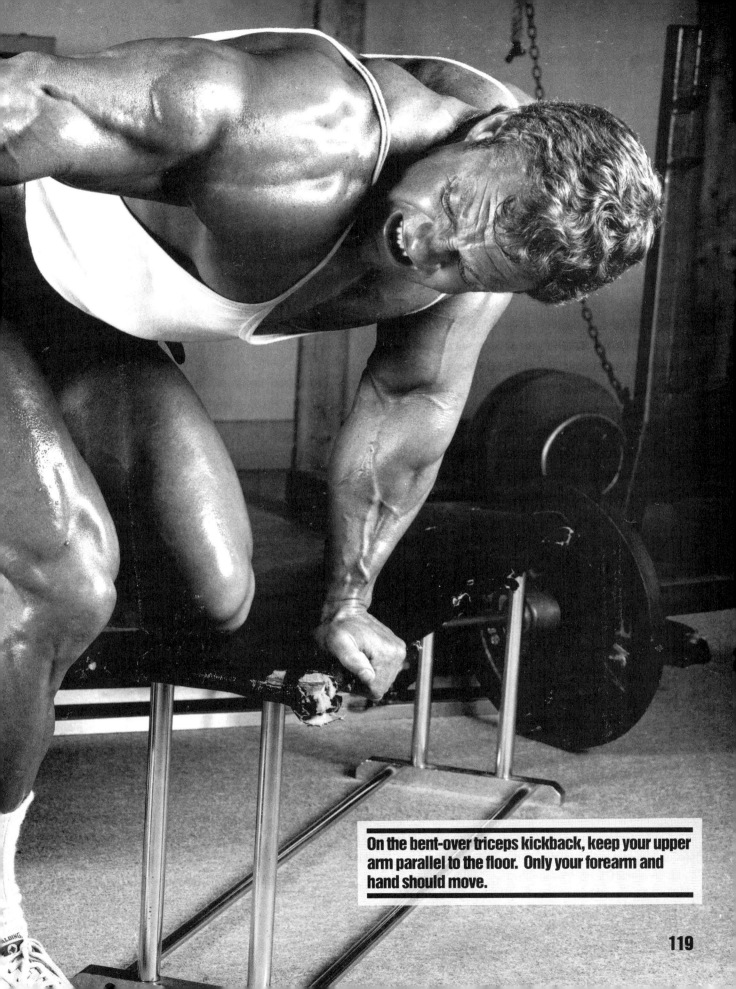

On the bent-over triceps kickback, keep your upper arm parallel to the floor. Only your forearm and hand should move.

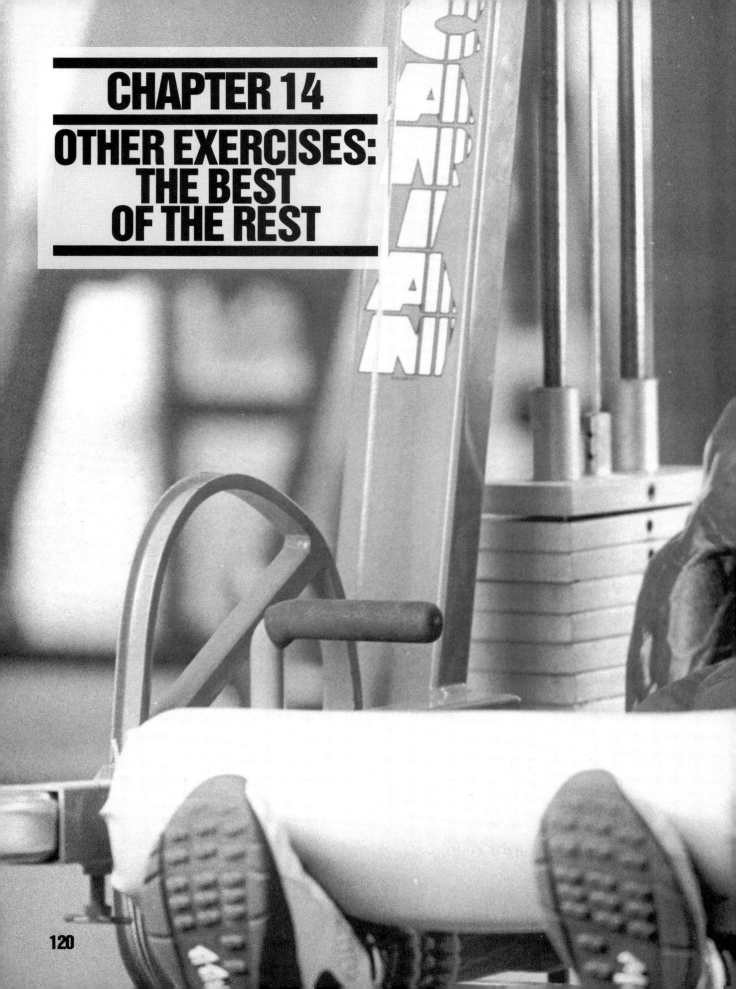

CHAPTER 14
OTHER EXERCISES: THE BEST OF THE REST

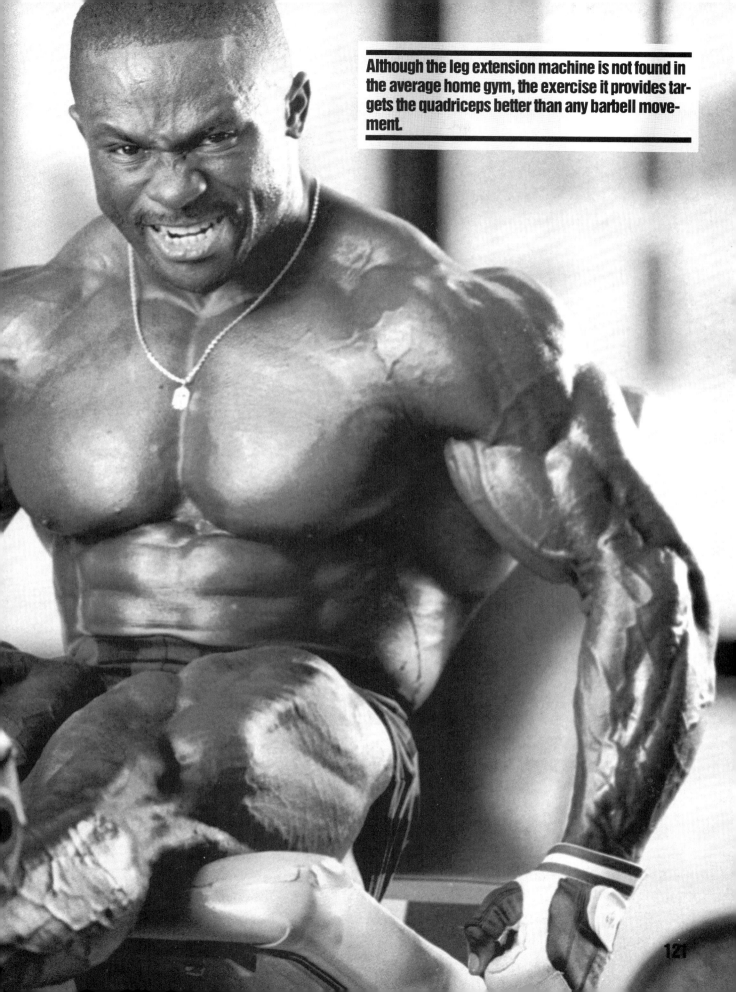

Although the leg extension machine is not found in the average home gym, the exercise it provides targets the quadriceps better than any barbell movement.

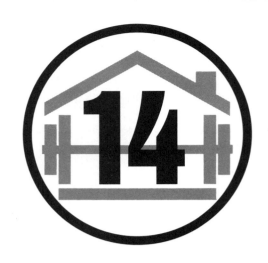

Before I get into the best of the other exercises, I'd like to supply you with a discussion of the exercises to avoid.

EXERCISES TO AVOID.

The following exercises are unsafe and should not be practiced:

- Power clean
- Clean-and-jerk
- Power snatch
- Snatch
- Lunge
- Jump squat
- Front squat
- Neck bridge

The power clean, clean-and-jerk, power snatch, and snatch are popular among Olympic weightlifters and necessary because these exercises are a part of their competition. The explosive nature of these lifts places tremendous forces on the involved muscles, connective tissues, and joints. Furthermore, these exercises all involve too much momentum to be effective and efficient muscle builders. Some football coaches recommend that their players do power cleans. They are of little value to a football player. Stay clear of these exercises or any other exercise that is done explosively.

The lunge with a barbell or dumbbells is another dangerous movement. Too much momentum is involved in stepping forward and backward with a heavy weight. Besides, the barbell squat is much safer and more productive.

The jump squat with a barbell or dumbbells is another unsafe exercise. Jumping by its very nature is explosive. Don't do it.

The front squat with a barbell, because of the placement of the bar across your clavicles, is uncomfortable and restraining. The barbell squat, again, is more productive.

The neck bridge is a favorite of many wrestlers. However, it places too much compression force on the cervical spine. Specifically designed neck machines by Nautilus or Hammer are recommended for the delicate neck muscles.

THE BEST OF THE REST

The following exercises require special equipment, or are not quite as productive as those discussed in Chapter 13. They still may be useful in your home-gym training.

- Seated calf raise (soleus)
- Lat machine pressdown (triceps)
- Leg extension (quadriceps)
- Lat machine pulldown (biceps and latissimus dorsi)
- Leg curl (hamstrings)
- Straddle lift (gluteals, quadriceps, and hamstrings)

The seated calf raise, leg extension, and leg curl are great exercises. But a specific machine is needed for each. If you have access to these machines, you'll certainly want to incorporate them into your routines.

The straddle lift, or Jefferson lift, is per-

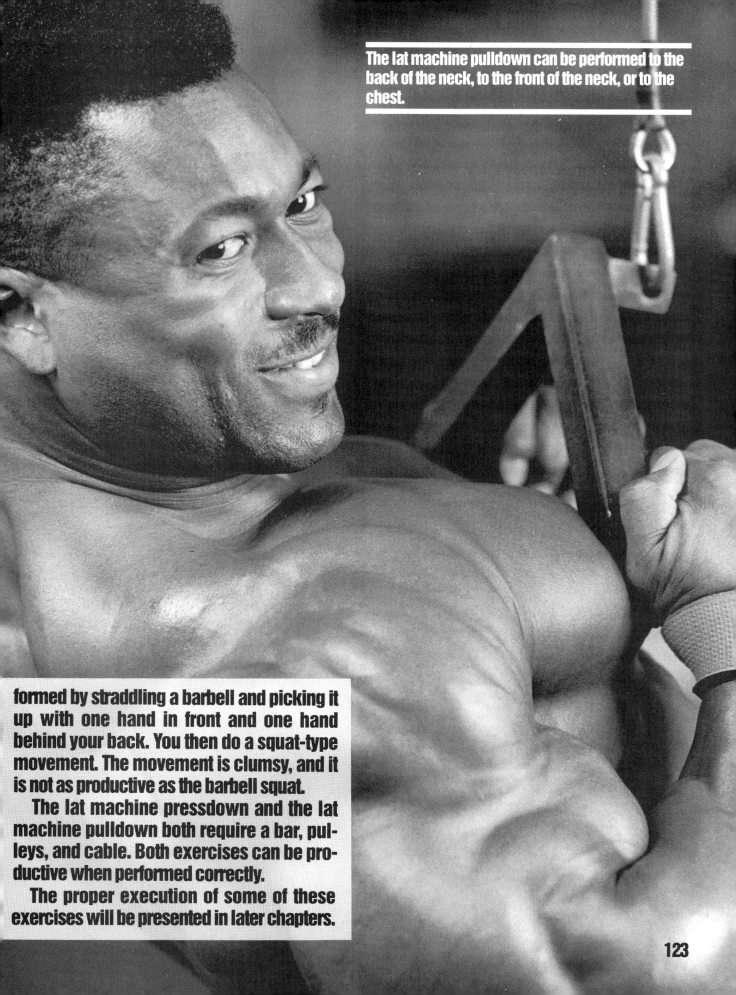

The lat machine pulldown can be performed to the back of the neck, to the front of the neck, or to the chest.

formed by straddling a barbell and picking it up with one hand in front and one hand behind your back. You then do a squat-type movement. The movement is clumsy, and it is not as productive as the barbell squat.

The lat machine pressdown and the lat machine pulldown both require a bar, pulleys, and cable. Both exercises can be productive when performed correctly.

The proper execution of some of these exercises will be presented in later chapters.

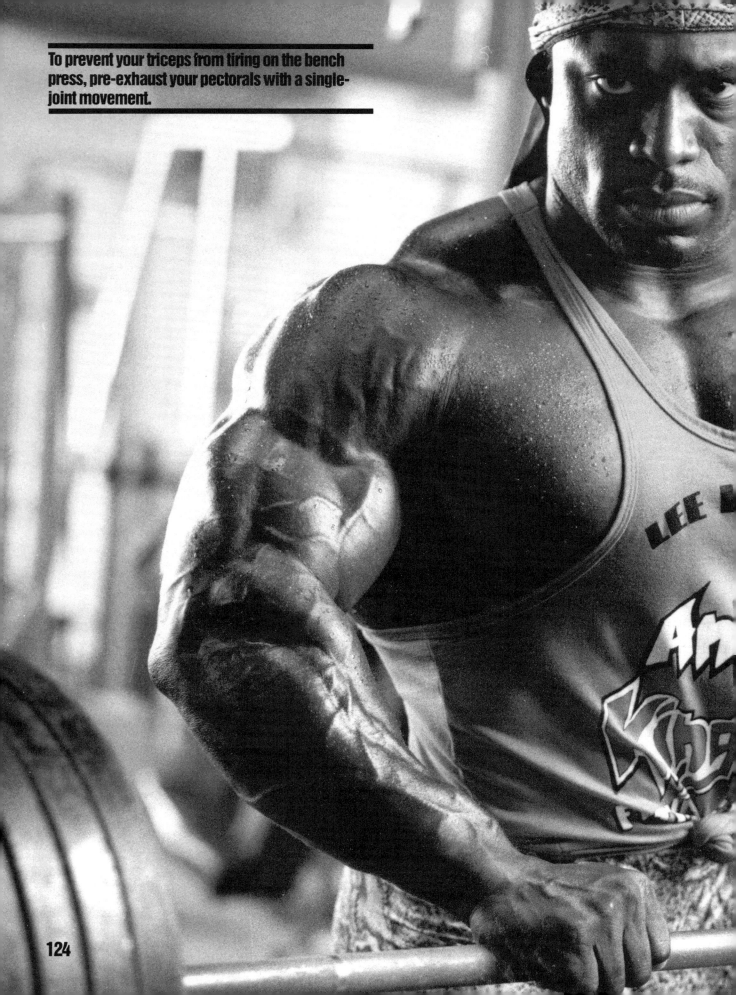

To prevent your triceps from tiring on the bench press, pre-exhaust your pectorals with a single-joint movement.

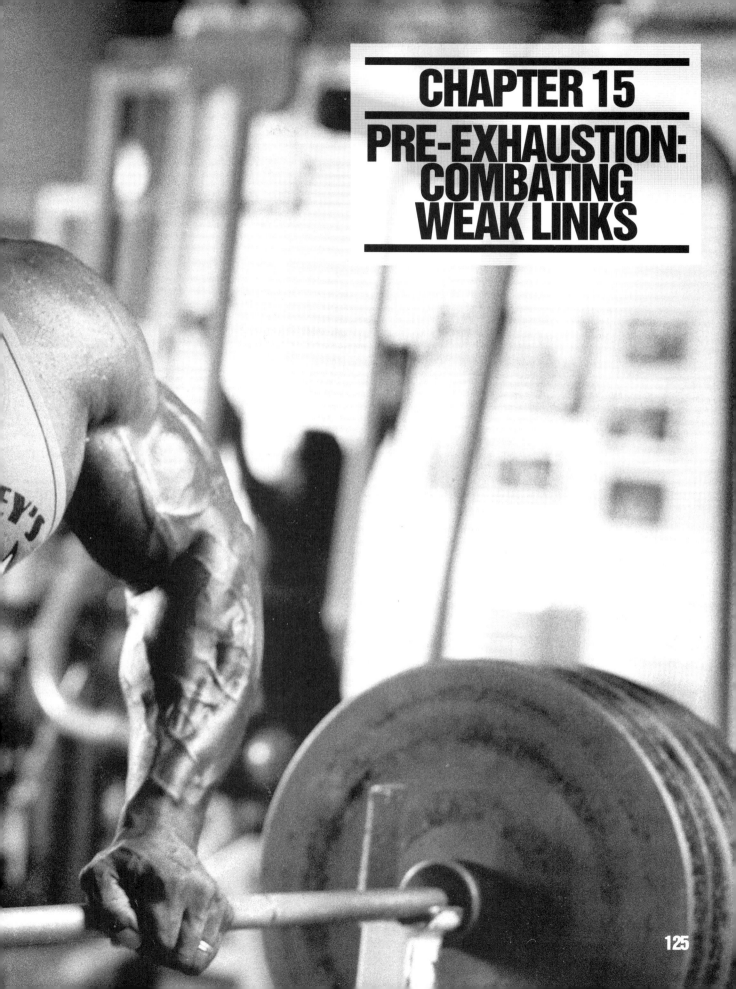

CHAPTER 15
PRE-EXHAUSTION: COMBATING WEAK LINKS

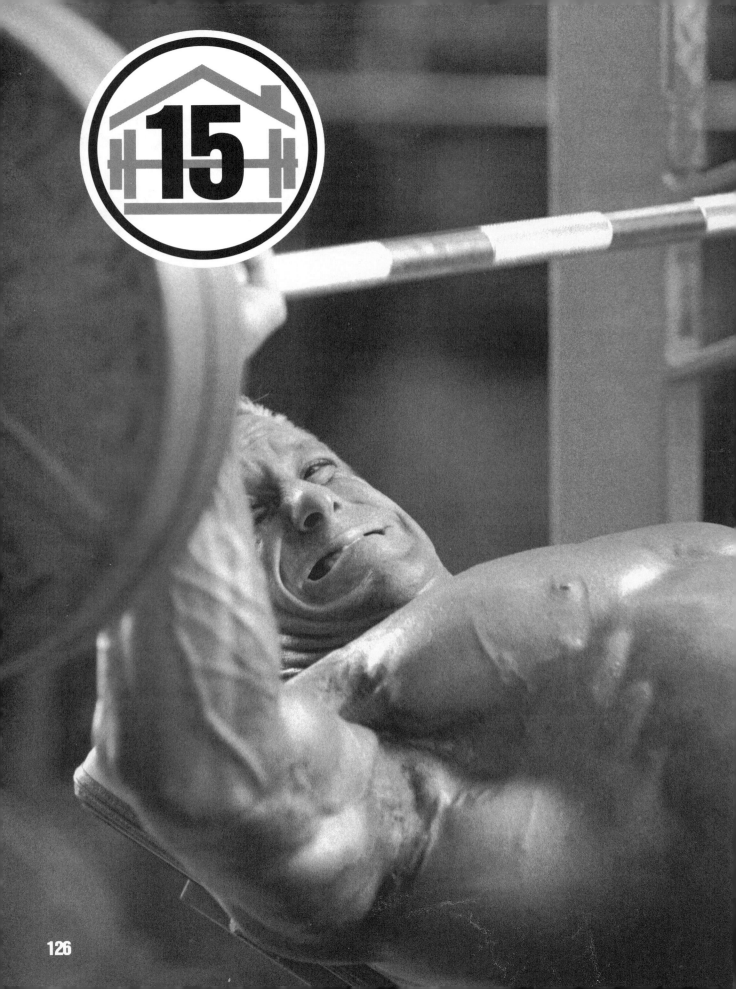

All multiple-joint exercises have a defect. The smaller, weaker muscles involved in the movement usually fatigue before significant growth stimulation occurs in the stronger muscles. The pre-exhaustion principle solves this problem.

WEAK LINKS

In the bench press, for example, your triceps tire before your larger, stronger pectorals do. You can combat this weak link by pre-exhausting your pectorals.

First, perform eight to twelve repetitions of the straight-armed fly with dumbbells, continuing until movement of the resistance is impossible. The straight-armed fly works your pectoralis major muscles without involving your triceps. Next, immediately do the bench press for as many repetitions as you can.

When you reach a point of failure on the bench press, it will not be because your triceps fatigued before your pectorals were worked properly. When you fail, it will be because your pectorals are exhausted. Your pectorals will now be stimulated to grow larger and stronger.

By pre-exhausting your pectoralis major muscles before doing the bench press, you have removed the weak link represented by triceps involvement in a multiple-joint pressing exercise.

NORMAL PRE-EXHAUSTION

Normal pre-exhaustion cycling combines

An understanding and application of the pre-exhaustion principle will boost your results from many multiple-joint exercises.

---

two exercises back-to-back. A single-joint movement is always followed by a multiple-joint movement. Examples of normal pre-exhaustion are the biceps curl and chin-up, the triceps extension and dip, the lateral raise and press behind neck, and the leg extension and squat.

A variation of this type of cycling is called double pre-exhaustion.

DOUBLE PRE-EXHAUSTION

This type of cycling involves three related exercises back-to-back. For example, you can do two single-joint movements back-to-back and follow them with a multiple-joint exercise. Or you can do a multiple-joint movement, then a single-joint exercise, and finally a multiple-joint movement.

Some examples of double pre-exhaustion are the following:

- Front raise, lateral raise, and overhead press
- Reverse curl, biceps curl, and lat machine pulldown
- Incline press, straight-armed fly, and dip
- Leg press, leg extension, and squat

THREE SECONDS OR LESS

On all pre-exhaustion cycles it is very important to move from one exercise to the next in three seconds or less. Taking longer than three seconds simply means that the involved muscles will have time to start recovering, and your subsequent growth stimulation will be less than it could have been. To combat this problem, arrange your exercise equipment so you can instantly move from one exercise to the next.

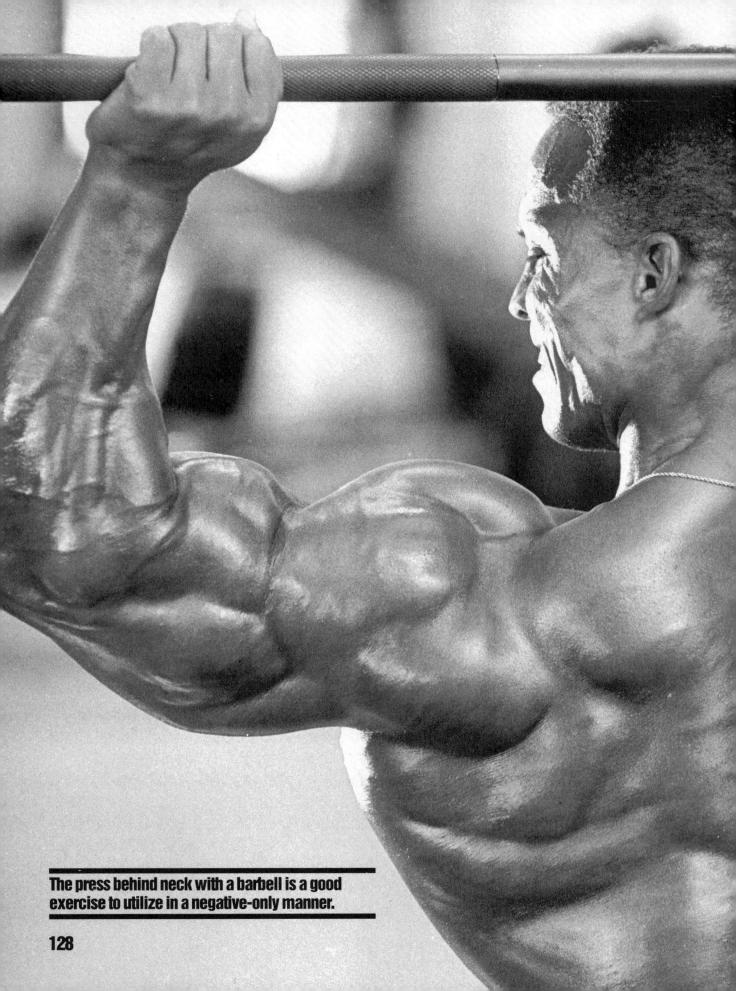

The press behind neck with a barbell is a good exercise to utilize in a negative-only manner.

CHAPTER 16
NEGATIVE-ONLY: CONTROLLED LOWERING

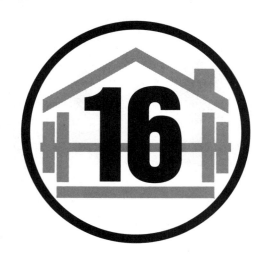

As you probably know, when you lift a weight your involved muscles contract or shorten. This shortening is called positive work. When you lower the weight, the same muscles extend or lengthen. This lengthening is termed negative work.

Research shows that your muscles are approximately 40 percent stronger during negative work than during positive work. In other words, if you can curl 100 pounds one time in a maximum effort, then you can lower under control 140 pounds. Research also reveals that lowering heavier weights than you can normally lift, called negative-only training, is very useful in increasing muscular size and strength.

In negative-only training, the weight, because it should be approximately 40 percent heavier than you normally handle for ten repetitions, must be lifted by one or two assistants. Then it's your job to slowly lower the resistance back to the bottom position. Your assistants lift the weight again, and you slowly lower it.

NEGATIVE HOW-TOS

The object of negative-only exercise is to lower the weight slowly, very slowly, in approximately ten seconds, but without interrupting the downward movement. At the start of a negative exercise, you should be able to stop the downward movement if you try. But do not try. After six or seven repetitions you should be unable to stop the downward movement no matter how hard you try. However, you should still be able to guide it into a slow, steady, smooth descent.

Finally, after two or three more repetitions you should find it impossible to stop the weight's downward acceleration. At that moment you should terminate the exercise.

Properly performed, negative-only exercise assures more complete involvement for the muscles, because the weight is never jerked or thrown. It always descends at a smooth, steady pace.

THE BEST NEGATIVE-ONLY MOVEMENTS

Having been involved with negative-only exercise for over twenty years, I find the following exercises most productive in a home-gym setting:

- Biceps curl, standing
- Bench press
- Press behind neck, seated
- Upright row
- Shoulder shrug
- Triceps extension, seated
- Leg extension (if machine is available)
- Leg curl (if machine is available)
- Chin-up
- Dip

The last two exercises, the chin-up and dip, are especially suitable for use in a neg-

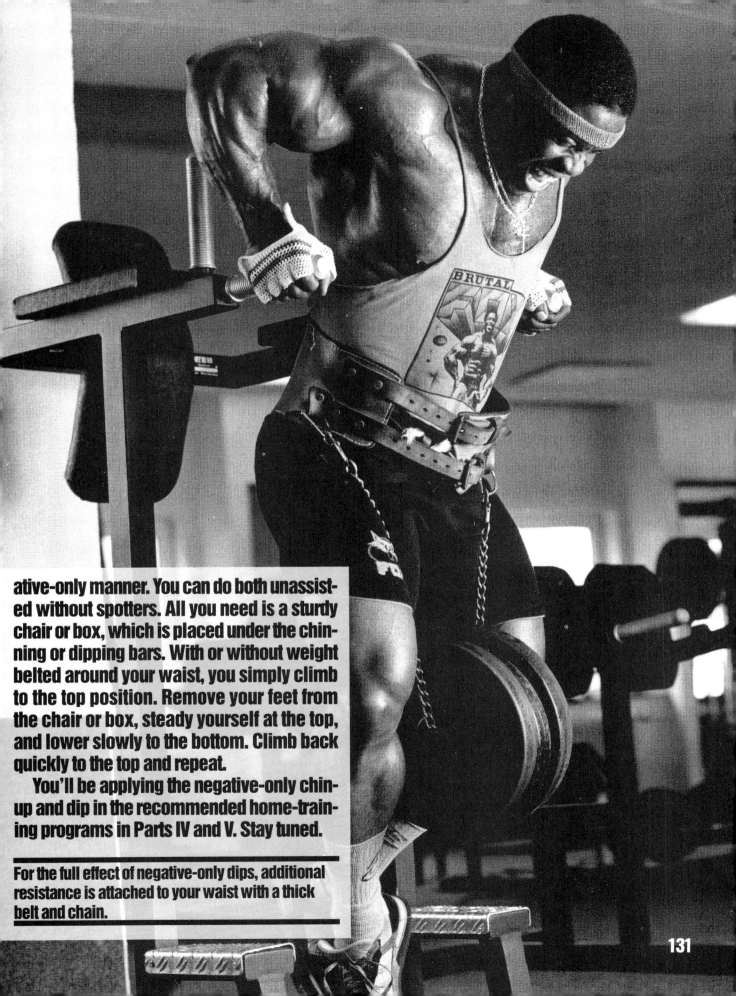

ative-only manner. You can do both unassist-
ed without spotters. All you need is a sturdy
chair or box, which is placed under the chinning or dipping bars. With or without weight
belted around your waist, you simply climb
to the top position. Remove your feet from
the chair or box, steady yourself at the top,
and lower slowly to the bottom. Climb back
quickly to the top and repeat.

You'll be applying the negative-only chin-
up and dip in the recommended home-train-
ing programs in Parts IV and V. Stay tuned.

For the full effect of negative-only dips, additional
resistance is attached to your waist with a thick
belt and chain.

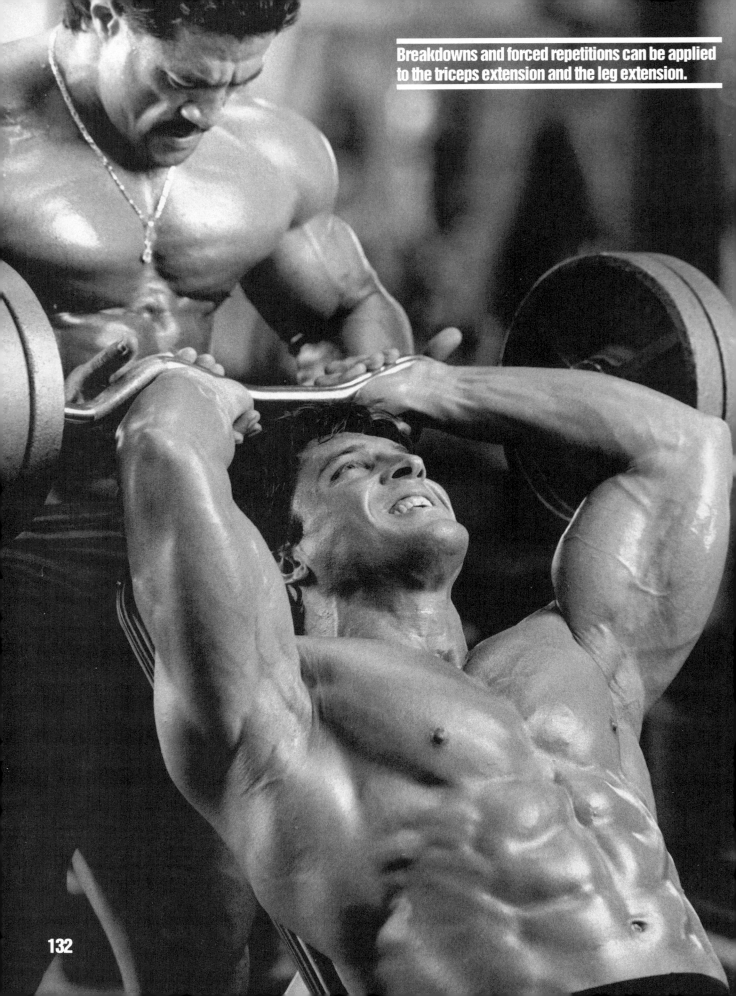

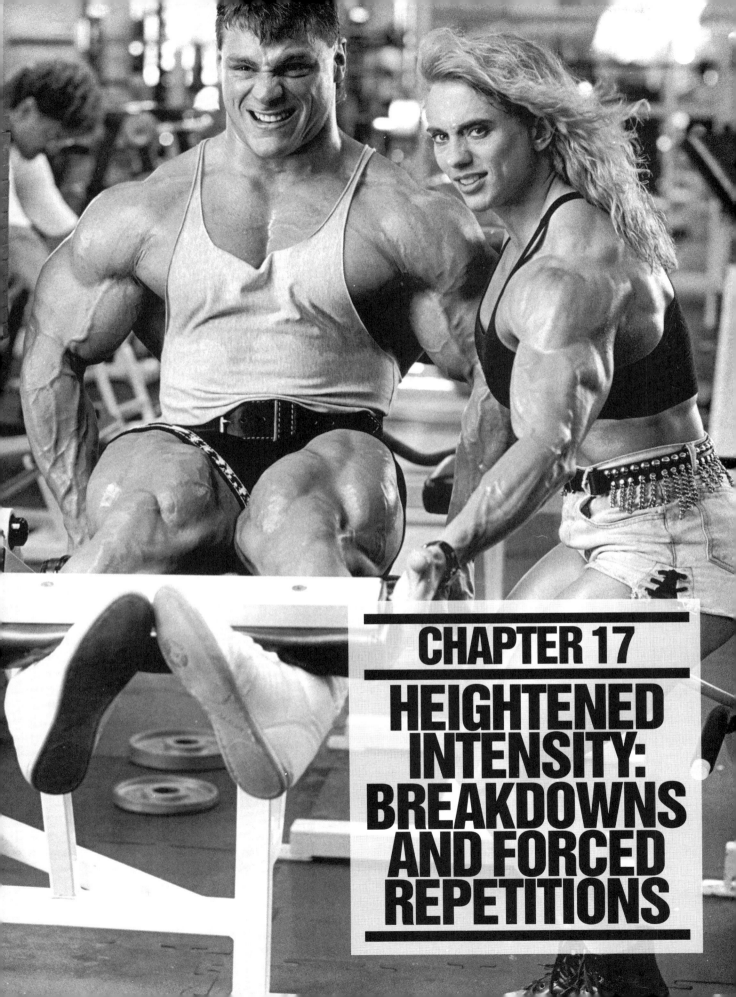

CHAPTER 17

HEIGHTENED INTENSITY: BREAKDOWNS AND FORCED REPETITIONS

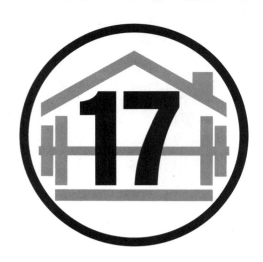

Pre-exhaustion cycles and negative-only exercises are ways to raise the intensity of your workouts. This chapter discusses two other techniques that heighten your intensity.

BREAKDOWNS

Breakdowns are an effective means for fatiguing additional muscle fibers at the end of a set. A set of ten repetitions usually fatigues approximately 20 percent of your muscle fibers. If your training partner immediately strips some small plates off either end of the barbell (approximately 10 percent of the weight on the bar), you can do a few more repetitions and thus fatigue more muscle fibers. In this manner, your involved muscles fail twice during this extended set.

You can apply breakdowns especially well to your smaller muscle groups because only a moderate amount of resistance is required for the barbell. Thus, it's simple to take off a five- or ten-pound plate from either side of the bar. With exercises for your larger muscle groups, two assistants are necessary to remove the heavier plates carefully and in a coordinated fashion.

FORCED REPETITIONS

Another way to heighten your intensity is by allowing your partner to give you forced repetitions. Instead of reducing the resistance once you reach failure, your partner assists you in doing a few more repetitions. Your partner provides just enough help for you to complete the positive phase of the exercise. Then you do the negative movement on your own. Three or four of these forced repetitions will involve more muscle fibers and stimulate greater muscular growth.

Too much of a good thing, however, can actually make too deep of an inroad into your starting level of strength. Doing so repeatedly with too many muscle groups can lead to overtraining.

Do not overdo forced repetitions or breakdowns. Use them sparingly. Use them wisely.

Shawn Ray prepares to do a set of dumbbell pullovers.

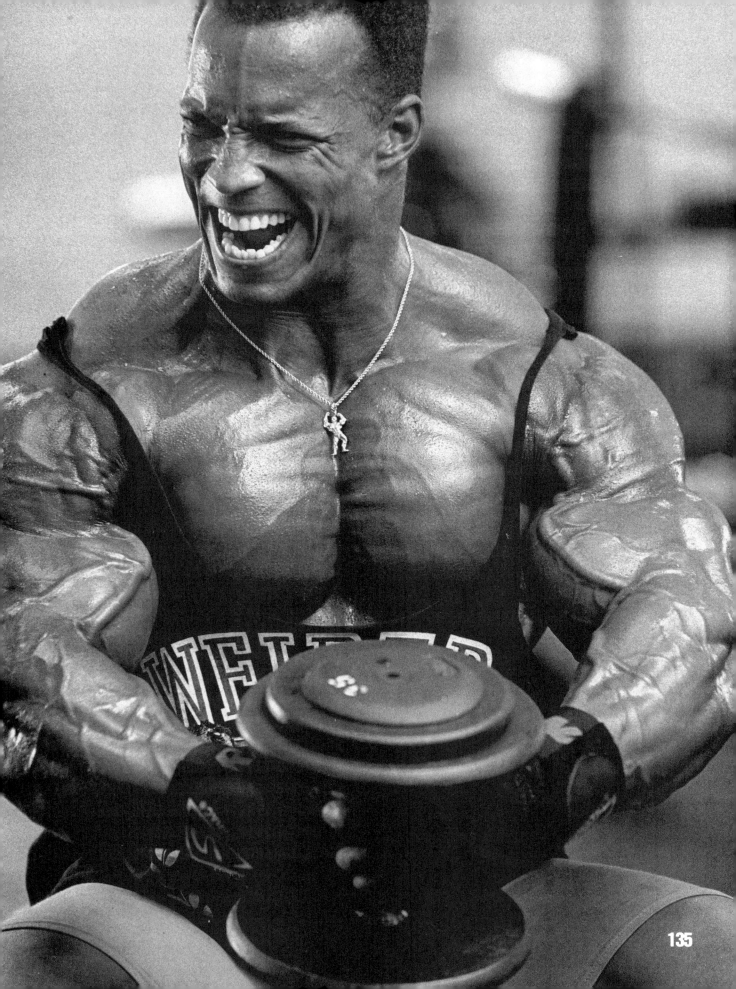

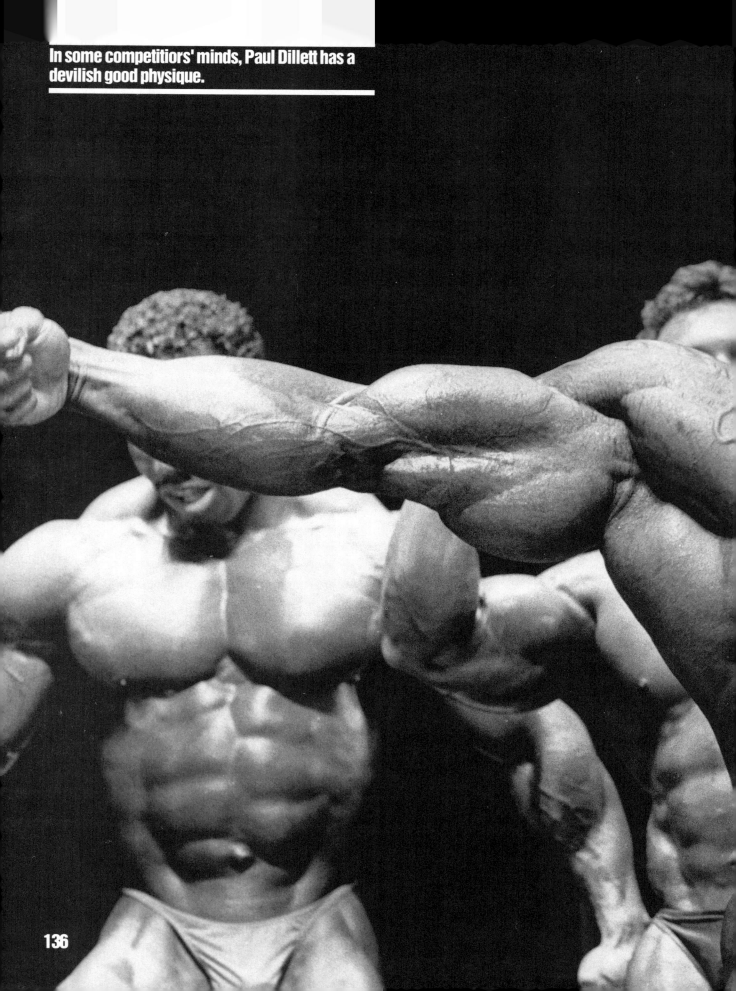

In some competitiors' minds, Paul Dillett has a devilish good physique.

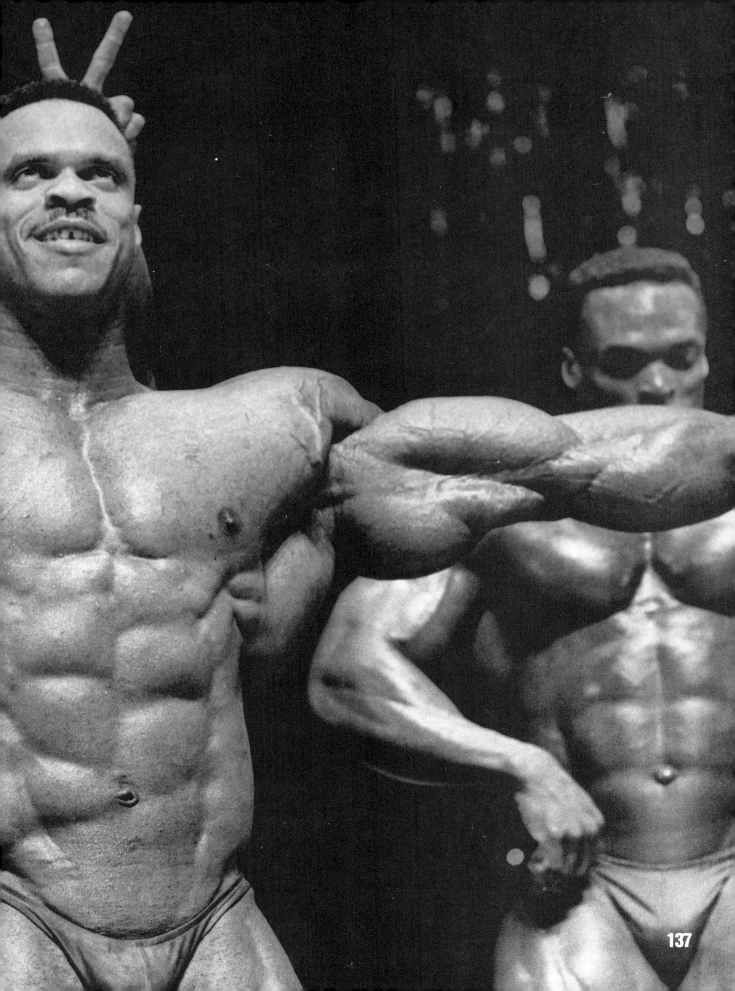

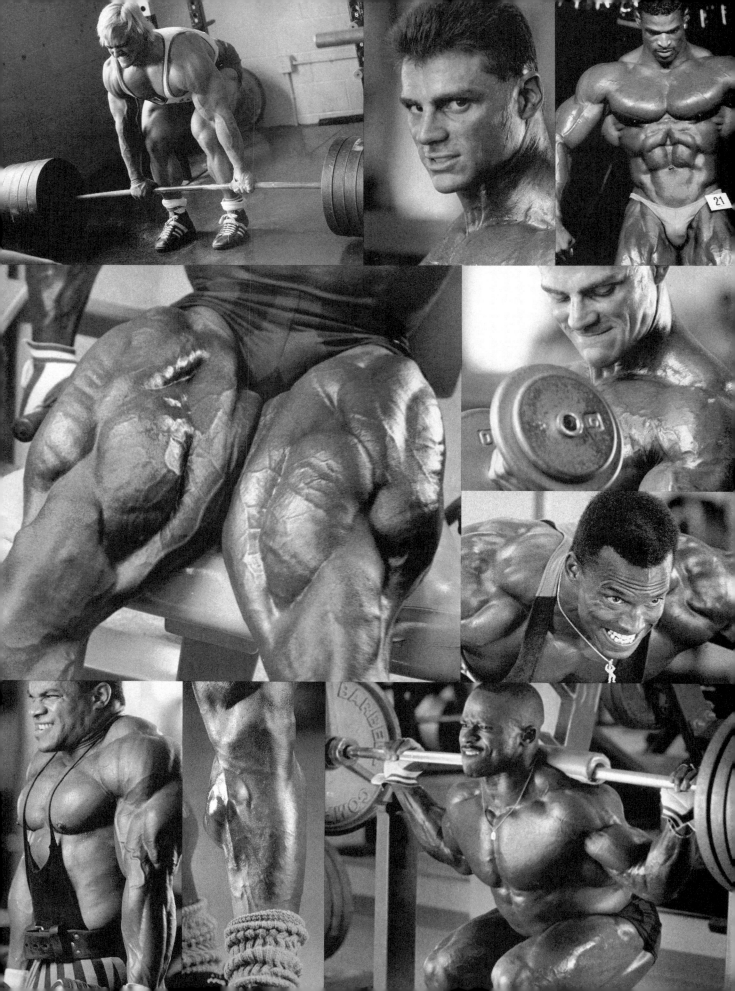

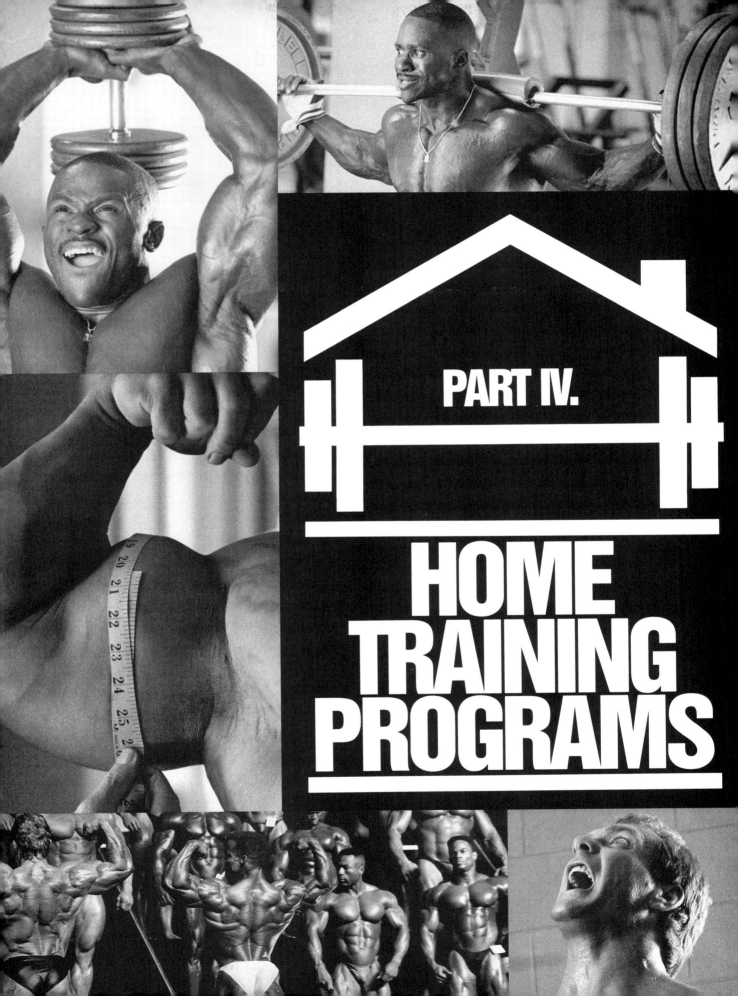

PART IV.

HOME TRAINING PROGRAMS

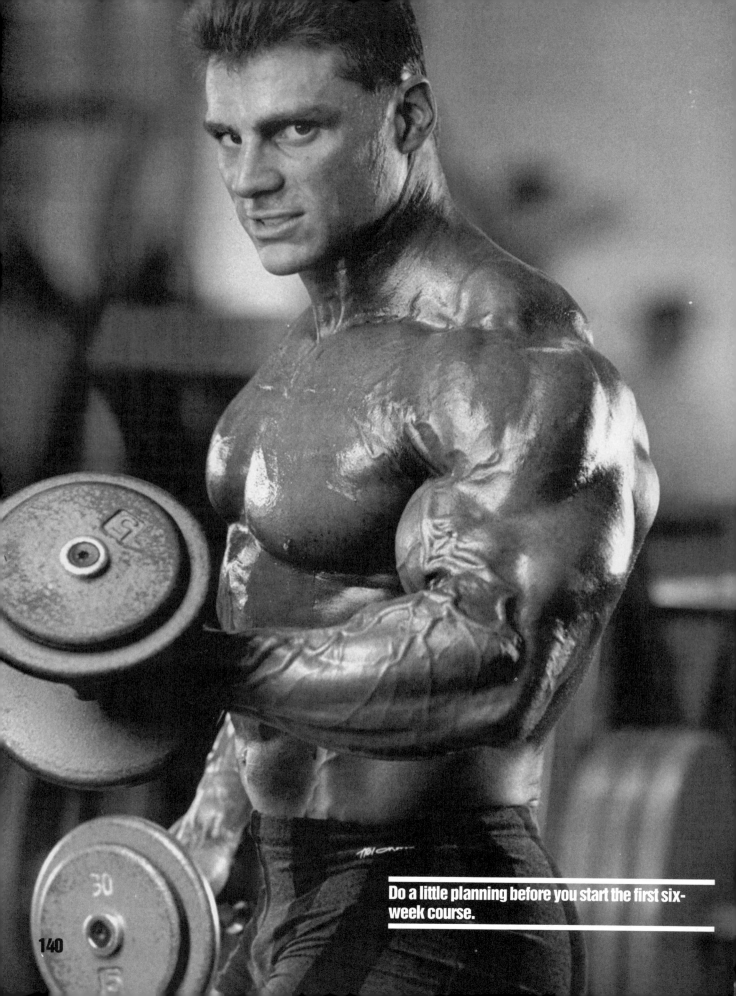

Do a little planning before you start the first six-week course.

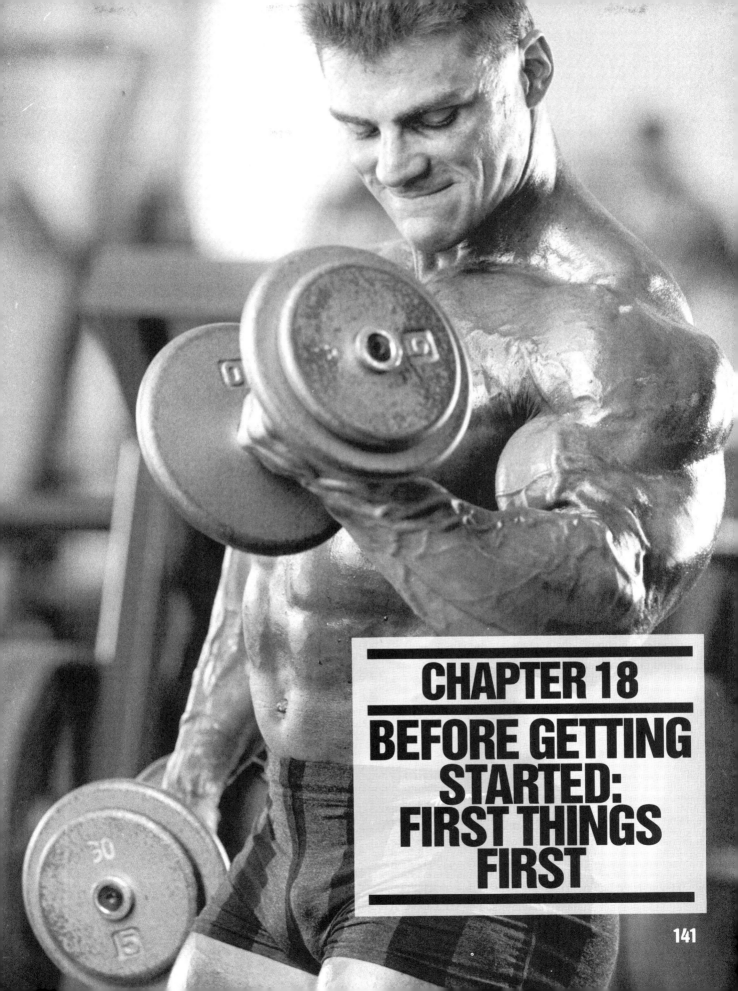

CHAPTER 18
BEFORE GETTING STARTED: FIRST THINGS FIRST

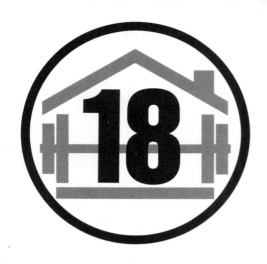

There are a few things you need to do before rushing into the training courses. Get your workout partner, and both of you take note of the following.

MEASUREMENTS

You'll want to keep accurate records of your body weight and body girths. This will allow you to better monitor your progress.

Record your body weight weekly, and do it at the same time. For example, record it immediately before your Monday workout.

Take your circumference measurements at the same time of day each time you do them. First thing in the morning is probably best. Do not pump your muscles; take the measurements cold. Avoid measuring yourself too often. Once every two to four weeks is about right.

Record measurements for your neck, forearms, upper arms, chest, waist, hips, thighs, and calves. Make a written note of the specific location you choose for each measurement. Precise descriptions of where and how to do this are described in two of my previous books: <u>Bigger Muscles in 42 Days</u> (Perigee Books, 1992) and <u>High-Intensity Strength Training</u> (Perigee Books, 1992). You can pick up a copy of either book at your local bookstore, or order one from the next-to-last page in this manual.

While your waist measurement and the thickness of a pinch of skin and fat on your midsection will provide a general guide on your percentage of body fat, you can be more accurate by using skinfold calipers. Follow the directions supplied with them carefully.

Another method of monitoring progress is before-and-after pictures. Have photographs taken every four to six weeks under the same conditions of angle, distance, lighting, attire, setting, poses, and film speed. Have the finished prints sized so your height is always the same. Being the same height in comparison prints allows your muscular progress to be seen at a glance.

WARMING UP

You do not have to go through an elaborate warm-up before your high-intensity training session. In fact, each exercise of eight to twelve repetitions has a built-in warm-up. Your initial six to seven repetitions are an effective warm-up for your last several repetitions, which are the hardest and the most productive.

Let's assume, for example, that you can complete twelve repetitions on the bench press in good form with one hundred pounds. If each repetition requires eight seconds, it will take approximately eighty to do ten repetitions. During this period, your triceps, deltoids, and pectoral muscles experience a very specific warm-up, and are well prepared for the final two repetitions. By the time your involved muscles exert maximum effort, they have had at least eighty seconds of progressively more difficult repetitions to stimulate the appropriate physiological adjustments.

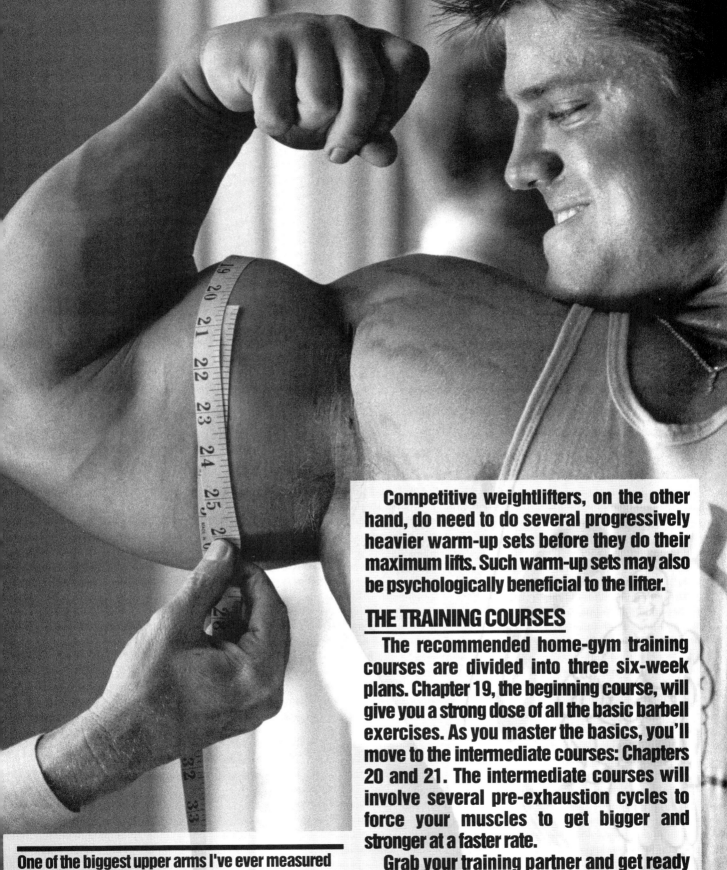

Competitive weightlifters, on the other hand, do need to do several progressively heavier warm-up sets before they do their maximum lifts. Such warm-up sets may also be psychologically beneficial to the lifter.

THE TRAINING COURSES

The recommended home-gym training courses are divided into three six-week plans. Chapter 19, the beginning course, will give you a strong dose of all the basic barbell exercises. As you master the basics, you'll move to the intermediate courses: Chapters 20 and 21. The intermediate courses will involve several pre-exhaustion cycles to force your muscles to get bigger and stronger at a faster rate.

Grab your training partner and get ready for some high-intensity muscle building. Get ready now!

One of the biggest upper arms I've ever measured belonged to Eddie Robinson. After a moderate workout, Eddie's arm measured 20 1/2 inches.

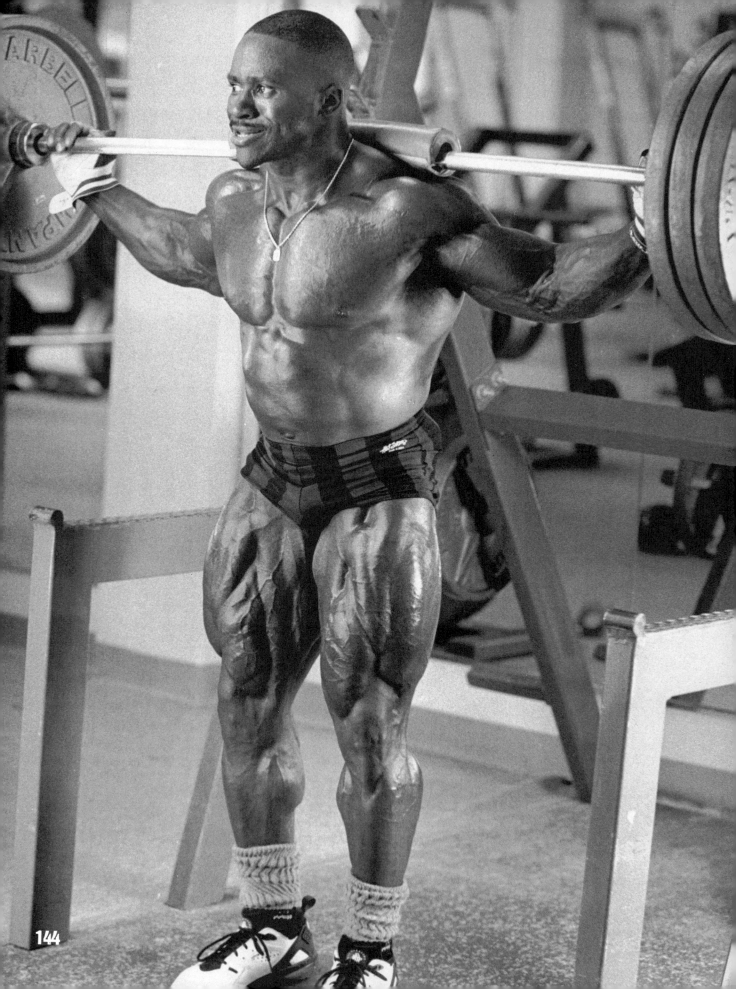

CHAPTER 19
BEGINNING COURSE: 1ST SIX WEEKS

The squat will tax your body from your neck down to your calves. Its overall growth effect is awesome.

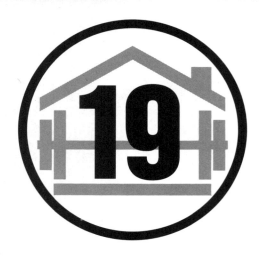

For the next six weeks, you'll be applying a high-intensity bodybuilding plan made up of primarily the basic barbell exercises. You will be training on a Monday-Wednesday-Friday schedule. You'll be doing one set of eight to twelve repetitions to momentary muscular failure.

You'll also want to make sure you are eating plenty of nutritious food, especially carbohydrates. A quick review of Chapter 3 will bolster your appetite.

Here's a brief exercise-by-exercise description of your beginning routine.

FIRST SIX WEEKS

1. Squat with barbell:

The loaded barbell is in the top position of the squat racks. Step under the barbell and place the bar behind your neck and across your shoulders. Stand erect and step back. Your feet are shoulder-width apart, and your head is up. Bend your hips and knees, and lower your buttocks until the backs of your thighs touch your calves. Do not bounce in and out of the bottom position. Return smoothly to the top position.

2. Straight-armed pullover with one dumbbell while lying crossways on a bench:

Lie down crossways on a bench with your shoulders in contact with the bench and your head and lower body relaxed and off the bench. A dumbbell, held on one end, is over your chest in a straight-armed manner. Take a deep breath and lower the dumbbell behind your head. Stretch and return the weight to the over-chest position. It is important to keep your arms straight during the movement and to emphasize the stretching of your torso when the dumbbell is behind your head. Repeat for eight to twelve repetitions.

3. Stiff-legged deadlift with barbell :

Grasp a barbell with an under-and-over grip. Your feet are under the bar. Lift the barbell to a standing position. Lower the bar for a comfortable stretch on your hamstrings. Keep a slight bend in your knees. Lift the weight smoothly back to the standing position and repeat.

4. Donkey calf raise:

You'll need a sturdy block of wood to stand on, a chair to lean against, and a training partner to sit across your hips. With your partner in position and the balls of your feet on the block of wood, lock your knees and keep them locked throughout the exercise. Raise and lower your heels slowly until momentary muscular failure. If you train alone, you can still perform this exercise by hanging weight around your hips with a weight belt.

5. Overhead press with barbell:

Clean a barbell to your shoulders. Your hands are shoulder-width apart. Press the bar smoothly over your head. Do not bend your knees or arch your back. Lower the barbell slowly to your shoulders. Repeat for maximum repetitions.

6. Bent-over row with barbell:

In a bent-over position, grasp a barbell

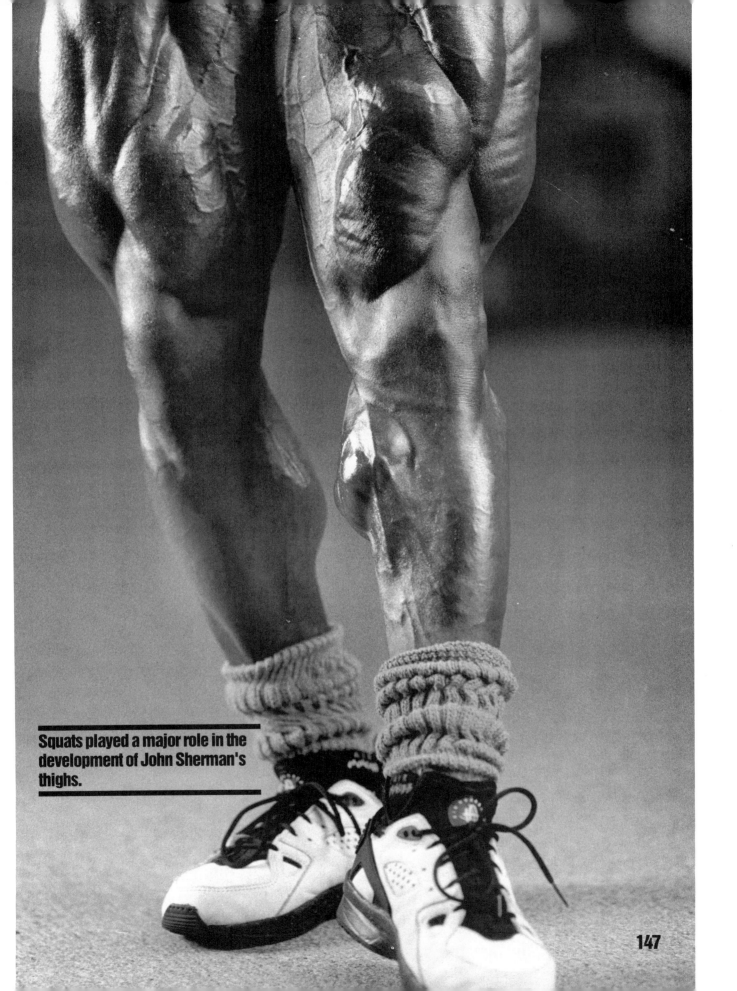

Squats played a major role in the development of John Sherman's thighs.

with a shoulder-width grip. Your torso is parallel to the floor. Pull the barbell upward until it touches your lower chest area. Pause. Return slowly to stretched position. Repeat.

7. Bench press with barbell:

It is best to use a standard bench with support racks for this exercise. Lie on your back and position your body under the racks and the supported barbell. Place your hands shoulder-width apart. Lift the barbell over your chest. Make sure your feet are flat on the floor in a stable position. Lower the barbell slowly to your chest. Press the barbell smoothly until your arms lock. Repeat for eight to twelve repetitions.

8. Shoulder shrug with barbell:

Grasp a barbell with an overhand grip and stand. Shrug your shoulders smoothly and try to touch your deltoids to your ears. Do not bend your elbows. Pause in the top position. Lower the barbell slowly and stretch. Repeat for maximum repetitions.

9. Dip:

Mount the parallel bars and lock your elbows. Bend your arms and lower your body for a comfortable stretch. Recover smoothly to the top position. Repeat until momentary muscular failure.

10. Chin-up:

Grasp a high horizontal bar with a palms-up grip and hang. Your hands are shoulder-width apart. Pull your body smoothly upward until your chin is over the bar. Lower your body smoothly to the hanging position. Repeat for as many repetitions as possible.

11. Press behind neck with barbell:

In a standing position, place a barbell behind your neck. Your hands are three inches wider apart than your shoulders. Press the barbell over your head smoothly. Lower the barbell slowly behind your neck. Do not bounce the bar off your shoulders. Keep the turnaround steady. Repeat.

12. Biceps curl with barbell:

Grasp a barbell with your palms up and your hands shoulder-width apart. Stand erect. While keeping your body straight, curl the barbell smoothly. Try to keep your elbows from moving forward or backward. Lower the bar smoothly. Repeat for eight to twelve repetitions.

13. Triceps extension with one dumbbell held in both hands:

Hold a dumbbell at one end with both hands. Press the dumbbell overhead. Your arms should be close to your ears. Bend your elbows and lower the dumbbell slowly behind your neck. Do not let your elbows drift; only your forearms and hands move. Extend the dumbbell back to the top position. Repeat.

14. Wrist curl with barbell:

Grasp a barbell with a palms-up grip. Anchor your forearms on your thighs and the backs of your hands against your knees, and sit on the end of a bench. Lean forward until the angle between your upper arms and forearms is less than ninety degrees. Curl your hands smoothly and contract your forearm muscles. Pause and lower the barbell slowly. Repeat the curling and lowering for maximum repetitions.

15. Reverse wrist curl:

Apply the same position as for the wrist curl, except use a palms-down grip. Reverse-curl the backs of your hands upward. Pause in the contracted position. Do

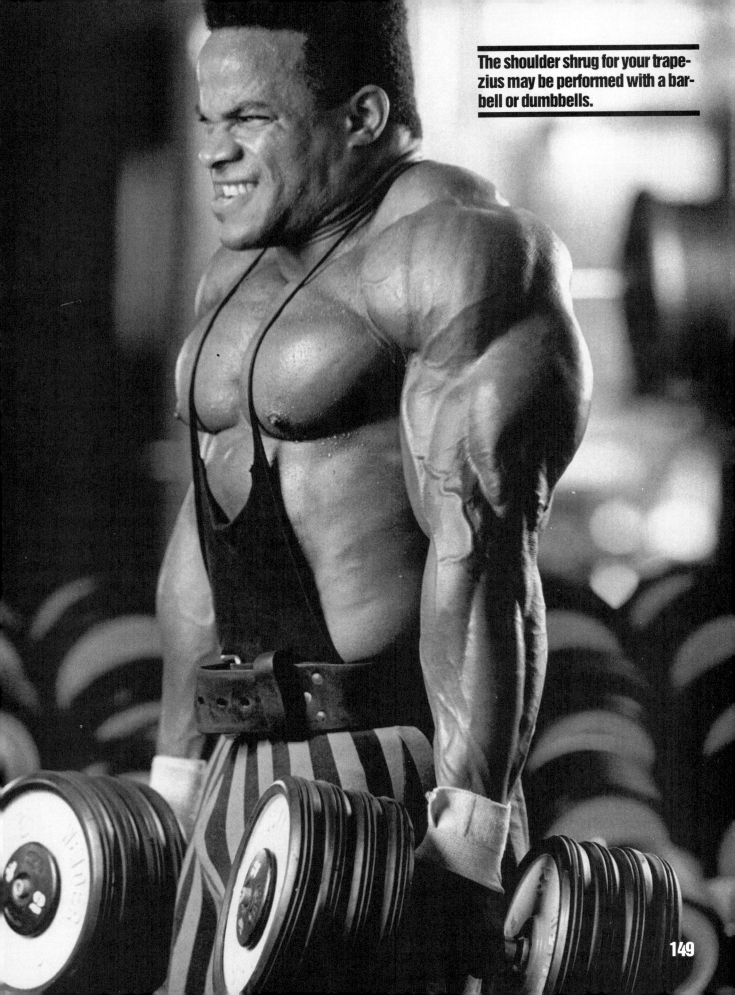

The shoulder shrug for your trapezius may be performed with a barbell or dumbbells.

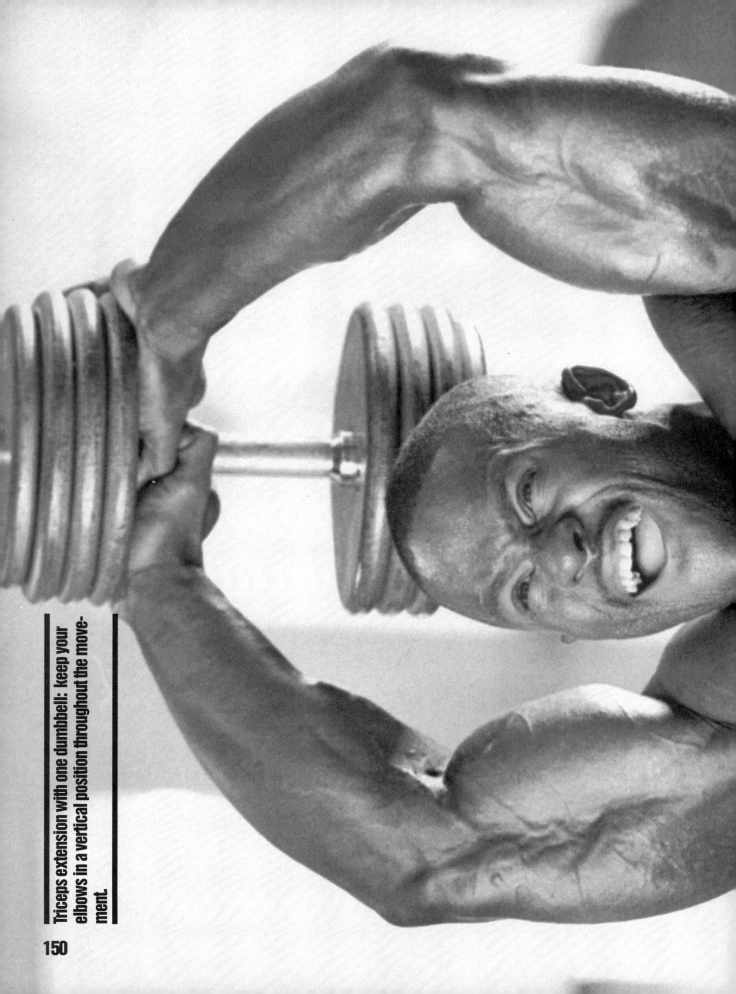

Triceps extension with one dumbbell: keep your elbows in a vertical position throughout the movement.

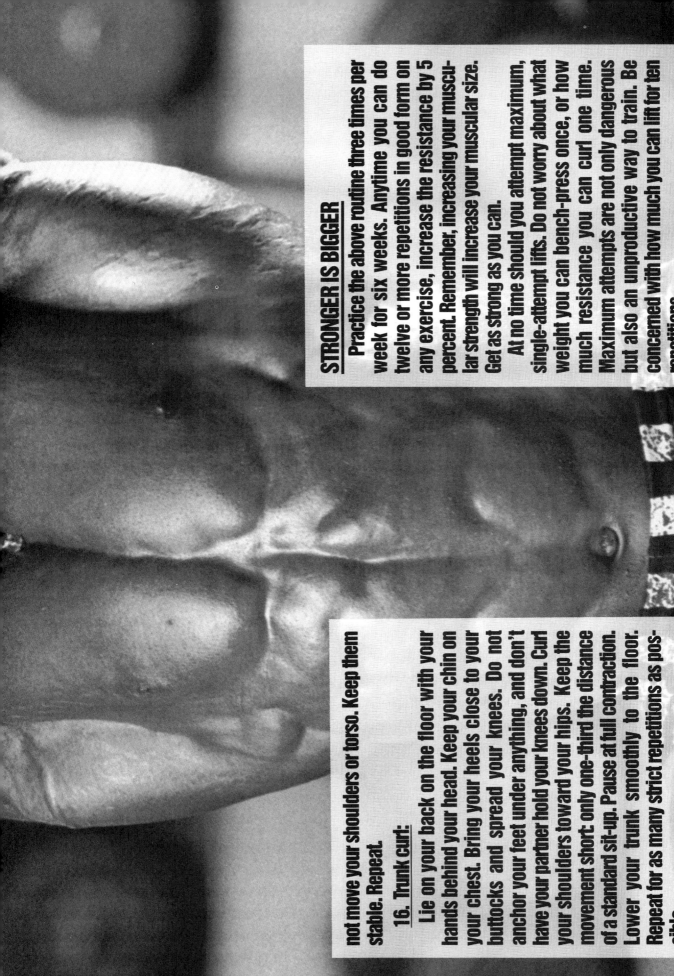

STRONGER IS BIGGER

Practice the above routine three times per week for six weeks. Anytime you can do twelve or more repetitions in good form on any exercise, increase the resistance by 5 percent. Remember, increasing your muscular strength will increase your muscular size. Get as strong as you can.

At no time should you attempt maximum, single-attempt lifts. Do not worry about what weight you can bench-press once, or how much resistance you can curl one time. Maximum attempts are not only dangerous but also an unproductive way to train. Be concerned with how much you can lift for ten repetitions.

not move your shoulders or torso. Keep them stable. Repeat.

16. Trunk curl:

Lie on your back on the floor with your hands behind your head. Keep your chin on your chest. Bring your heels close to your buttocks and spread your knees. Do not anchor your feet under anything, and don't have your partner hold your knees down. Curl your shoulders toward your hips. Keep the movement short only one-third the distance of a standard sit-up. Pause at full contraction. Lower your trunk smoothly to the floor. Repeat for as many strict repetitions as possible.

CHAPTER 20
INTERMEDIATE COURSE: 2ND SIX WEEKS

In doing the deadlift, keep the movement smooth and steady.

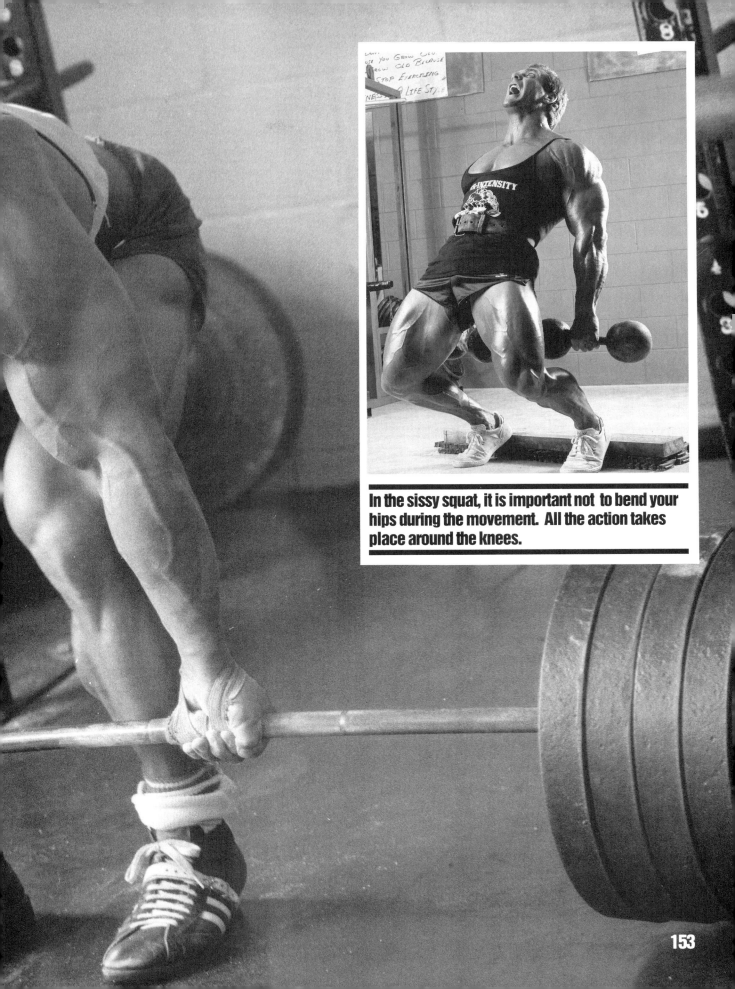

In the sissy squat, it is important not to bend your hips during the movement. All the action takes place around the knees.

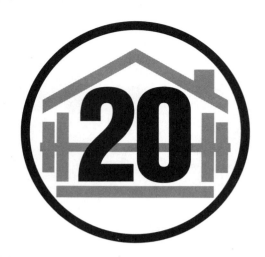

One thing that will help you make better progress during the second six weeks is to eat some carbohydrates immediately after your workout. Research shows that fatigued muscles are most responsive to energy storage within the initial thirty minutes following a high-intensity training session. What works best for many of my athletes is one or two bananas washed down with a pint of chocolate milk. Try these after your next workout.

The second six weeks also involves sixteen exercises, some of which are different than those of the first six weeks.

SECOND SIX WEEKS

1. Squat with barbell:

Continue your squatting as before. Your legs should be getting larger and stronger.

2. Straight-armed pullover with one dumbbell while lying crossways on a bench:

Squats followed by pullovers have a stimulating effect on expanding your rib cage. Breathe deeply as you stretch and contract on this result-producing movement.

3. Sissy squat:

Your body weight is all the resistance you'll need on this exercise for a while. Place your heels shoulder-width apart on a three-inch-thick block of wood. The idea now is to bend your knees while keeping your thighs and torso on the same plane. As you lean back you'll be in a limbo dance position at the bottom. Return smoothly to the top, but do not straighten your knees completely. Start another repetition immediately. You'll feel this interesting exercise entirely in your quadriceps. Eventually, when you require more resistance than your body weight, you can hold a dumbbell in each hand.

4. Hack squat with barbell:

Roll a barbell slightly behind the three-inch block of wood. Place your heels shoulder-width apart on the wood and go into a squat position. Reach down with your hands and grasp the barbell behind your heels with a palms-down grip. Keep your back upright as you straighten your knees and hips. When you reach a standing position, the barbell is behind your hips. Bend your knees and hips while holding the barbell behind your hips and do squats in this manner for as many repetitions as possible. On the final repetition, place the barbell on the floor.

5. Bent-armed pullover with barbell:

Lie on a bench with your head barely off the edge. Anchor your feet securely underneath. Have your training partner hand you the loaded barbell. Your hands are twelve inches apart as the barbell rests across your chest. Move the bar just over your face and head, and smoothly try to touch the floor. Don't straighten your arms; keep them bent. Stretch in the bottom position and smoothly pull the barbell above your face to your chest. Repeat for eight to twelve repetitions.

6. Lateral raise with dumbbells:

Grasp a dumbbell in each hand and stand.

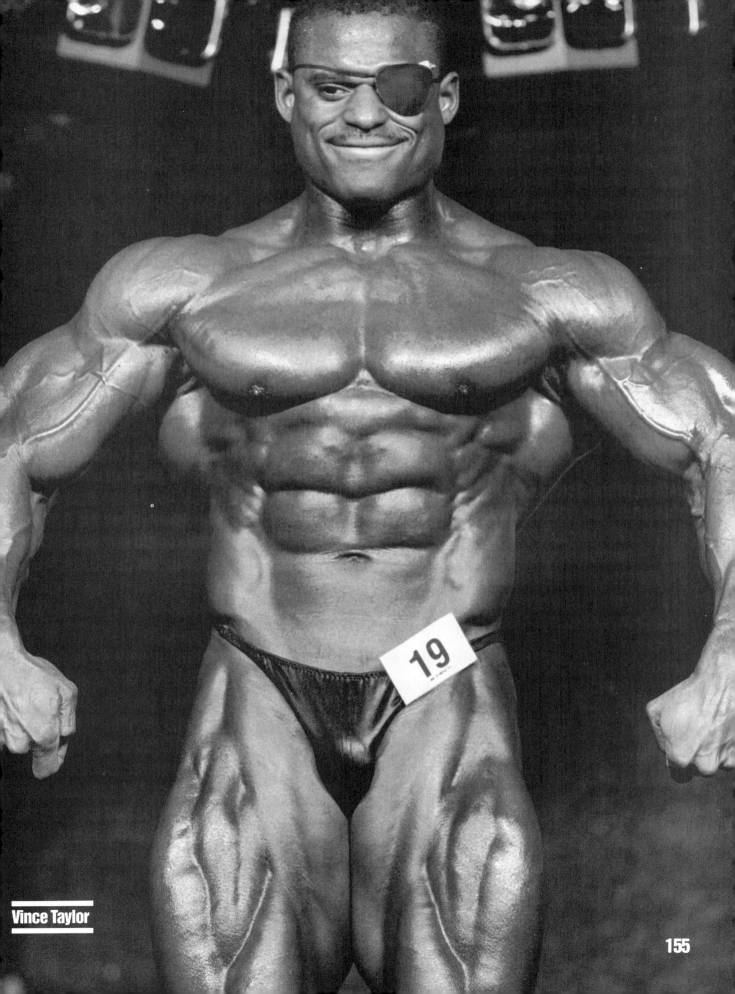

Vince Taylor

Lock your elbows and wrists and keep them stable throughout the exercise. All the action occurs around your shoulder joints. Raise your arms sideways smoothly. Pause briefly when the dumbbells are slightly above the horizontal position. Make sure your palms are facing down. Lower slowly to your sides. Repeat the raising and lowering for maximum repetitions.

7. Overhead press with barbell:

Keep the pressing movements smooth and steady. Do not rest in the top or bottom position. Grind out as many repetitions as you can without cheating.

8. Behind-neck chin-up:

Hang from a horizontal bar with your hands spaced approximately twelve inches wider than your shoulders. Use an overhand grip. Pull your body up and forward until the bar touches behind your neck. Pause at the top and lower slowly to the bottom position. Repeat for as many repetitions as possible.

9. Shoulder shrug with barbell:

Strive to get as much range of movement as you can from each repetition.

10. Upright row with barbell:

Grasp a barbell with a palms-down grip and stand. There is about six inches of space between your index fingers, and the barbell is leaning against your thighs. Pull the barbell upward along the front of your body until your hands almost touch your neck. Make sure your elbows stay above your hands. Lower the bar smoothly back to your thighs. Repeat for maximum repetitions.

11. Triceps extension with one dumbbell held in both hands:

Work your triceps intensely for the required repetitions.

12. Biceps curl with barbell:

Keep your repetitions strict to guarantee thorough involvement of your biceps.

13. Wrist curl with barbell:

Perform this exercise very slowly for best results.

14. Reverse curl with barbell:

Take a shoulder-width palms-down grip on a barbell and stand with your arms at your sides. Anchor your elbows against your waist throughout the movement. Reverse-curl the barbell smoothly. Pause in the top position, but do not move your elbows forward. Lower the bar slowly. Repeat for eight to twelve repetitions.

15. Reverse trunk curl:

Lie faceup on the floor with your hands at your hips. Bring your thighs to your chest so your knees and hips are in a flexed position. Curl your hips toward your chest by lifting your buttocks and lower back off the floor. At the same time that you lift your buttocks, you must counterbalance your body by pushing down on the floor with your hands and arms. Pause briefly in the top position. Lower your hips slowly to the floor. Repeat the curling and lowering for maximum repetitions.

16. Deadlift with barbell:

Grasp a barbell with an under-and-over grip. Your feet are under the bar. Bend your knees as you lift the barbell to a standing position. Lower the barbell to the floor by bending your hips and knees. Repeat the smooth lifting and lowering.

THE MOST PRODUCTIVE BARBELL EXERCISES

This intermediate course starts with the squat and ends with the deadlift. The squat

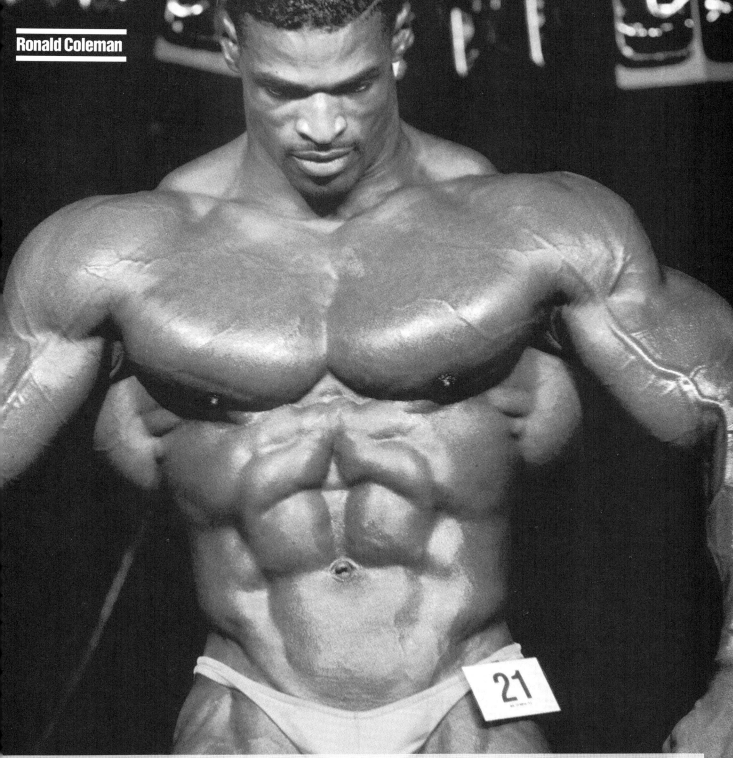

Ronald Coleman

and the deadlift are the two most productive barbell exercises that you can do to stimulate overall muscular size and strength. It's because these exercises demand such intense work, and affect such a large amount of muscle, that they are so effective at producing results.

Development of your hip, thigh, and back musculature is the base for massive growth throughout your body. For each workout during the second six weeks, give the squat and the deadlift your supreme effort. With dedicated work, you'll be ready to progress to the third six weeks.

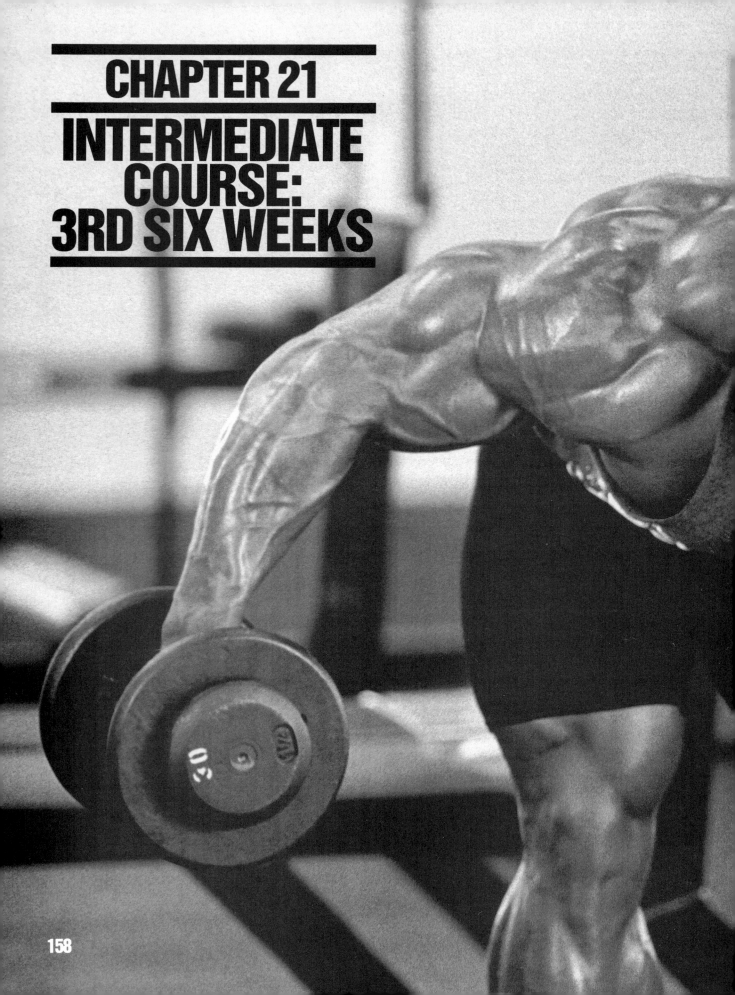

CHAPTER 21
INTERMEDIATE COURSE:
3RD SIX WEEKS

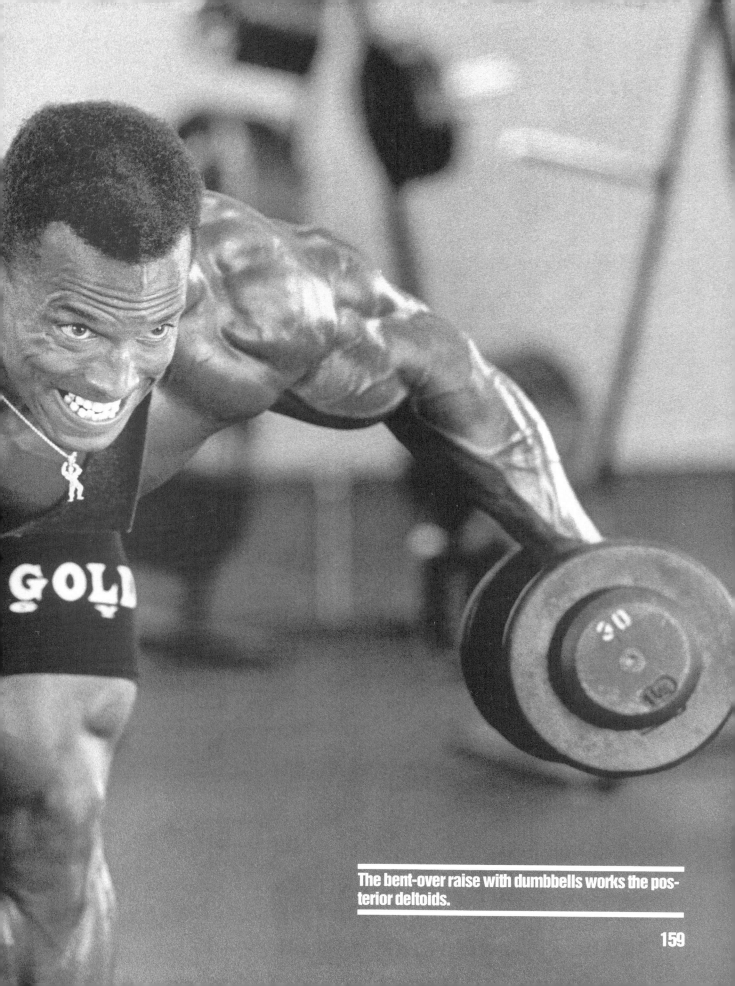

The bent-over raise with dumbbells works the posterior deltoids.

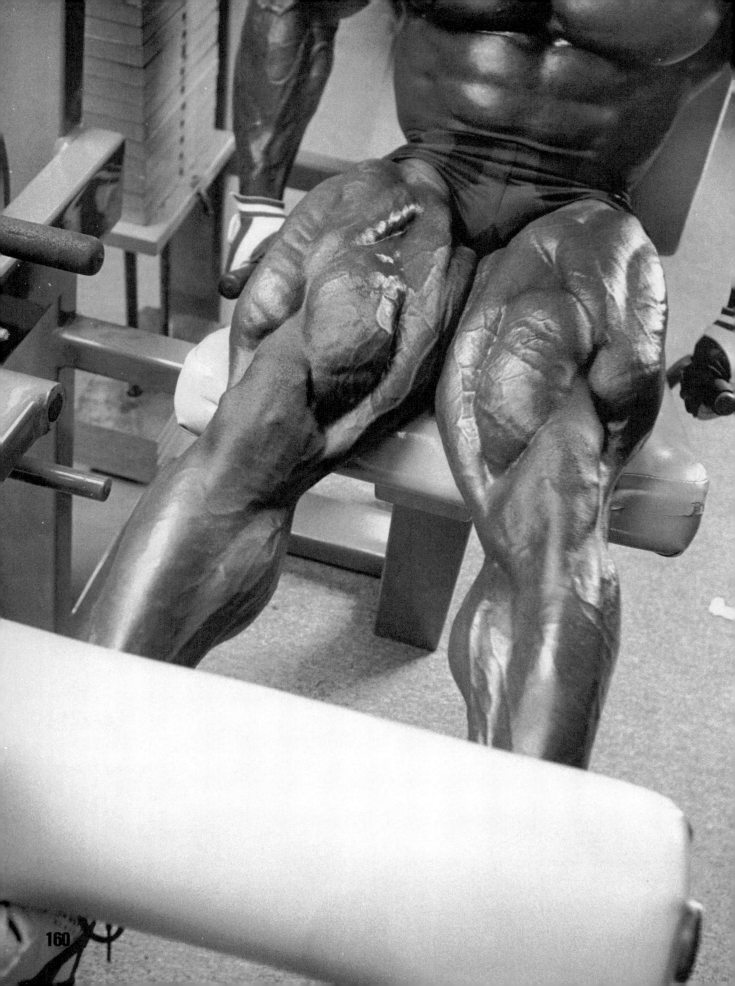

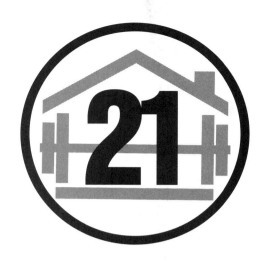

You've been training in the high-intensity fashion for twelve weeks. You've been working hard doing sixteen exercises three times per week. And you should be getting bigger and stronger by the day.

As you get stronger, however, you are capable of making deeper demands on your body's ability to recover. Your recovery ability does not increase in proportion to your body's capacity for strength. To continue to get bigger and stronger at a consistent rate, you must do less overall exercise.

During the third six weeks, you will still train three times per week. Every other workout, however, you'll reduce the exercises from sixteen to twelve. In other words, on Monday and Friday of the first week you'll do sixteen exercises. On Wednesday, you'll do only twelve. On Monday and Friday of the second week, you do twelve exercises. On Wednesday, you perform sixteen. You should continue in this manner for the entire six weeks.

On your twelve-exercise days, you will eliminate the leg extension, squat, straight-

---

For best results on the leg extension, pause briefly in the top position.

armed fly, and bench press. Here is a description of all the exercises in the routine.

THIRD SIX WEEKS

1. Leg curl machine:

If you don't have access to a leg curl machine, you'll have to use the stiff-legged deadlift instead. Lie facedown on the leg curl machine with your knees on the pad edge closest to the movement arm. Hook your heels under the roller pads. Make certain your knees are in line with the axis of rotation of the machine. Curl your heels smoothly and try to touch the roller pads to your buttocks. Pause briefly in the top position. Lower slowly for a comfortable stretch. Repeat for eight to twelve repetitions.

2. Leg extension machine:

If a leg extension machine is not available, substitute the sissy squat. Sit in the machine and place your feet behind the bottom roller pads. If possible, align the axis of rotation of the movement arm with your knees. Lean back and stabilize your upper body by grasping the side of the machine. Straighten your legs smoothly and ease into the fully contracted top position. Pause briefly. Lower the weight slowly and repeat until failure.

3. Squat with barbell:

Unrack the bar and start doing repetitions smoothly. Think positive. They do seem to get somewhat easier after the third repetition, at least until the ninth or tenth. Try to get twelve repetitions, if possible.

4. Donkey calf raise:

Be sure to go all the way up and all the way down on this excellent movement for your lower legs.

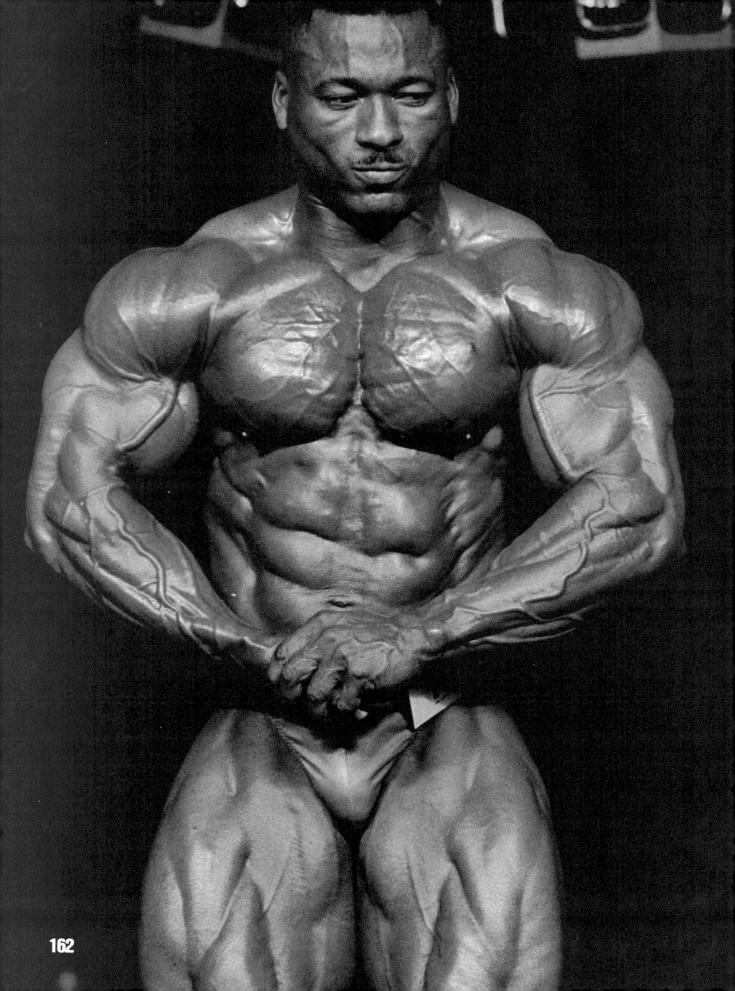

5. Chin-up:

Do as many repetitions as you can of the chin-up with a palms-up grip.

6. Straight-armed fly with dumbbells:

Grasp two dumbbells, lie back on a flat bench, and extend both arms over your chest. Your palms are facing each other while holding the dumbbells. Keep your elbows locked as you lower the dumbbells out to your sides as low as comfortably possible. Return the dumbbells smoothly along the same arcs to the top position. Repeat for eight to twelve repetitions.

7. Bench press with barbell:

Do each repetition in a smooth, steady style.

8. Bent-over row with barbell:

Keep the repetitions strict and remember to pause briefly in the top position.

9. Press behind neck with barbell:

For best results, make this movement continuous: no pausing at the top and no pausing at the bottom.

10. Shoulder shrug with barbell:

Work on raising your shoulders up to your ears.

11. Dip on parallel bars:

Be sure to get a full range of movement on all your dips.

12. Biceps curl with barbell:

Try to relax your face as you do the curls and you'll get more growth stimulation on your biceps.

13. Bent-over triceps kickback with dumbbells:

Henderson Thorne displays striking mass and hardness.

Take a dumbbell in each hand and bend at the waist until your torso is parallel to the floor. Keep your upper arms next to your sides. Extend your forearms back and contract your triceps intensely. Pause briefly in the contracted position. Lower the dumbbells, but keep your upper arms stationary. Repeat for as many repetitions as possible.

14. Bent-over raise with dumbbells:

With a pair of light dumbbells in your hands, bend over until your torso is parallel to the floor. Let the dumbbells hang. Raise the dumbbells smoothly backward as far as possible. Do not bend your elbows. Keep them straight throughout the movement. Pause in the top position. Lower and repeat for eight to twelve repetitions.

15. Wrist curl with barbell:

Grip the barbell intensely as you flex and extend your wrists.

16. Trunk curl:

Your abdominals will feel this exercise if you focus on moving smoothly and slowly on each repetition.

SIMPLE, INFREQUENT TRAINING

"The appalling irony of modern bodybuilding," Stuart McRobert writes in Brawn, "is that the training methods appropriate to only a small minority of bodybuilders are given massive promotion, while the training methods most appropriate to the masses are largely hidden from the very people who need them the most."

McRobert is referring to the split routines of two days on and one day off, three days on and two days off, six days on and one day off. Often, promotion is given to twice-a-day workouts and twelve or more sets per body part of three different exercises.

Such high-volume training works consistently only for the genetically gifted athlete who is probably on one or more anabolic drugs. It doesn't produce results for average bodybuilders, the hard-gainers. In fact, it has an appalling failure rate.

What's needed are simple and infrequent routines.

That's what the first, second, and third six-week courses in this book provide: simple, three-times-per-week training. Remember, once you stimulate growth, your body must have adequate rest and recovery to grow.

Practice these courses exactly as described and your muscles are guaranteed to get larger and stronger. In three to four months, you should add 100 pounds to your squat, 75 pounds to your bench press, and 35 pounds to your biceps curl. As soon as you accomplish these goals, you'll be ready for the advanced, specialized routines in Part V.

It is important that you master the basics before you specialize.

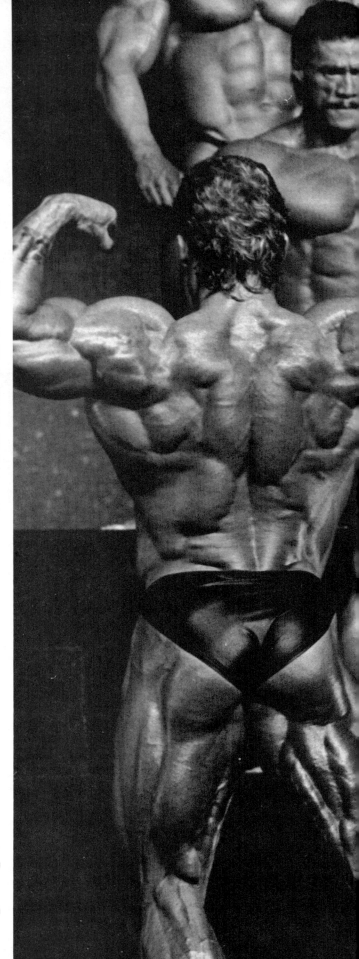

Dorian Yates and Shawn Ray contract their backsides.

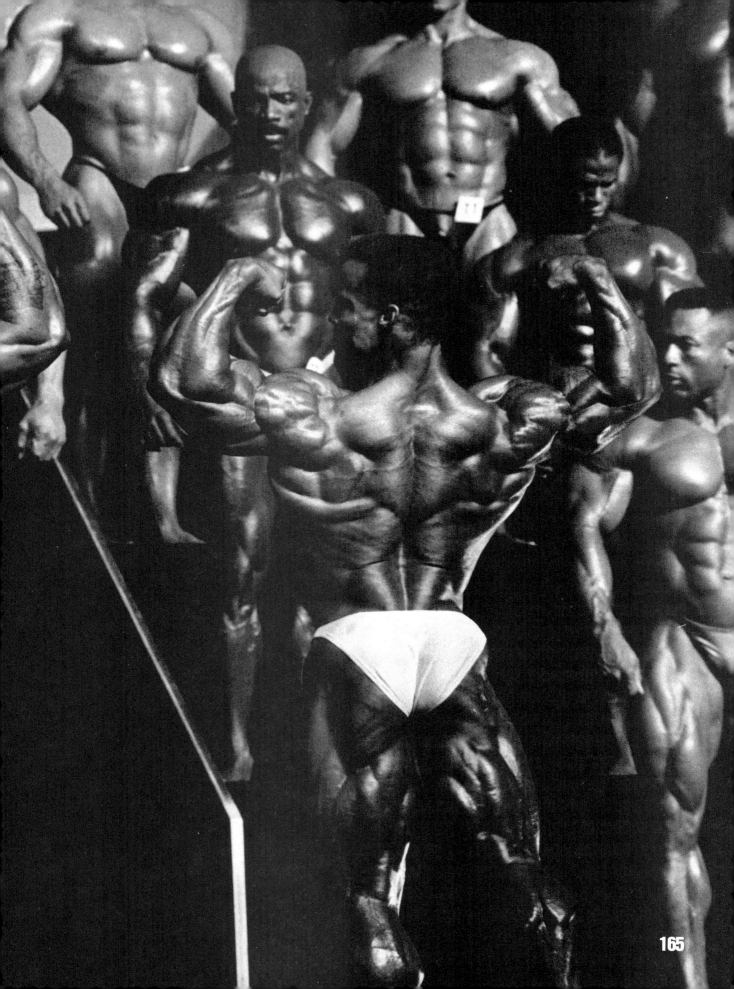

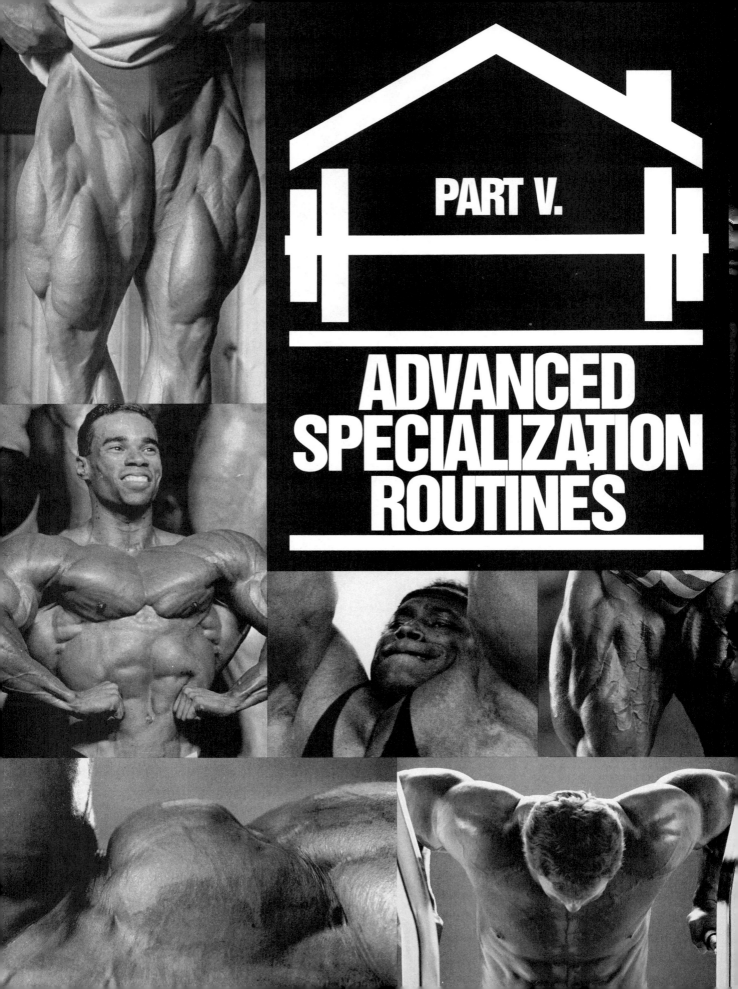

PART V.

ADVANCED SPECIALIZATION ROUTINES

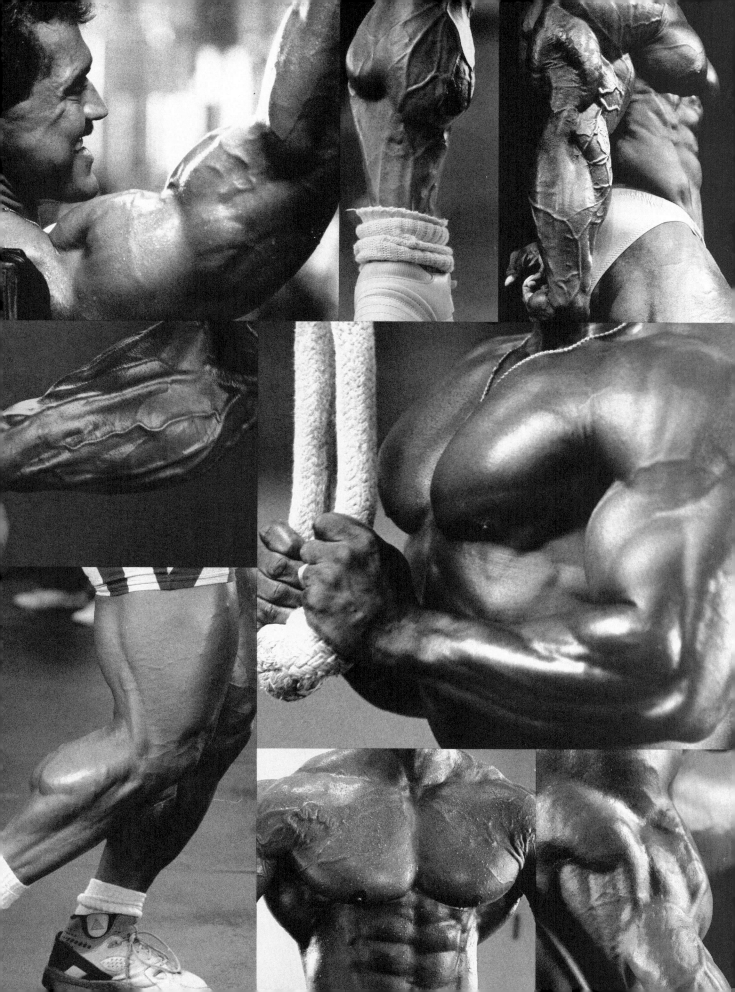

CHAPTER 22
THIGHS: STRONG AND SEPARATED

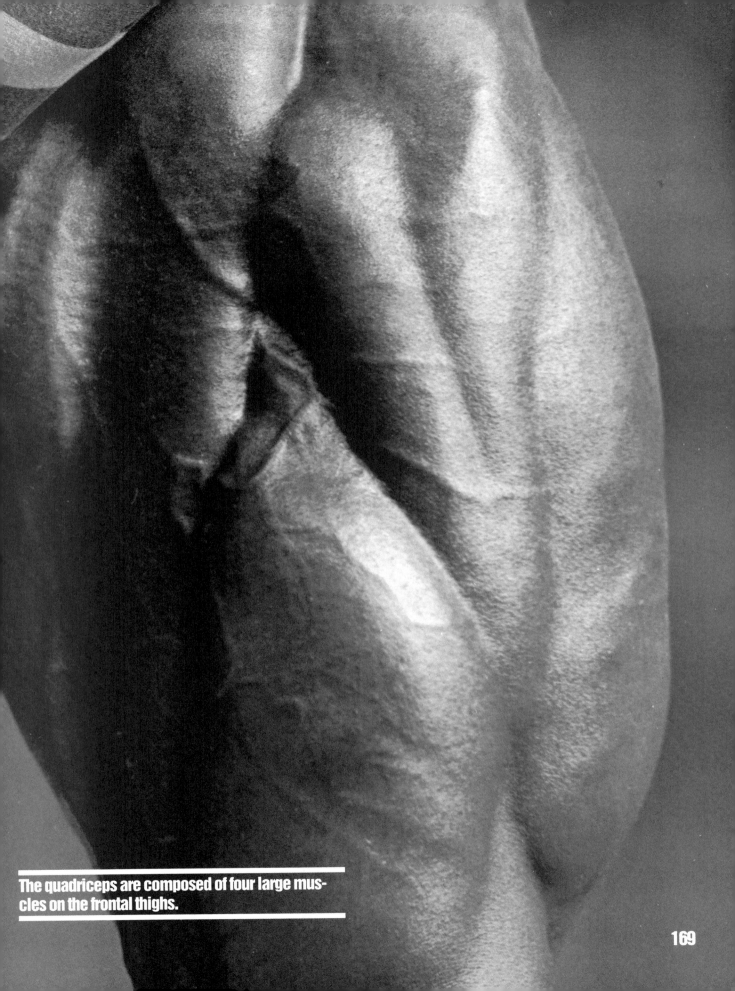

The quadriceps are composed of four large muscles on the frontal thighs.

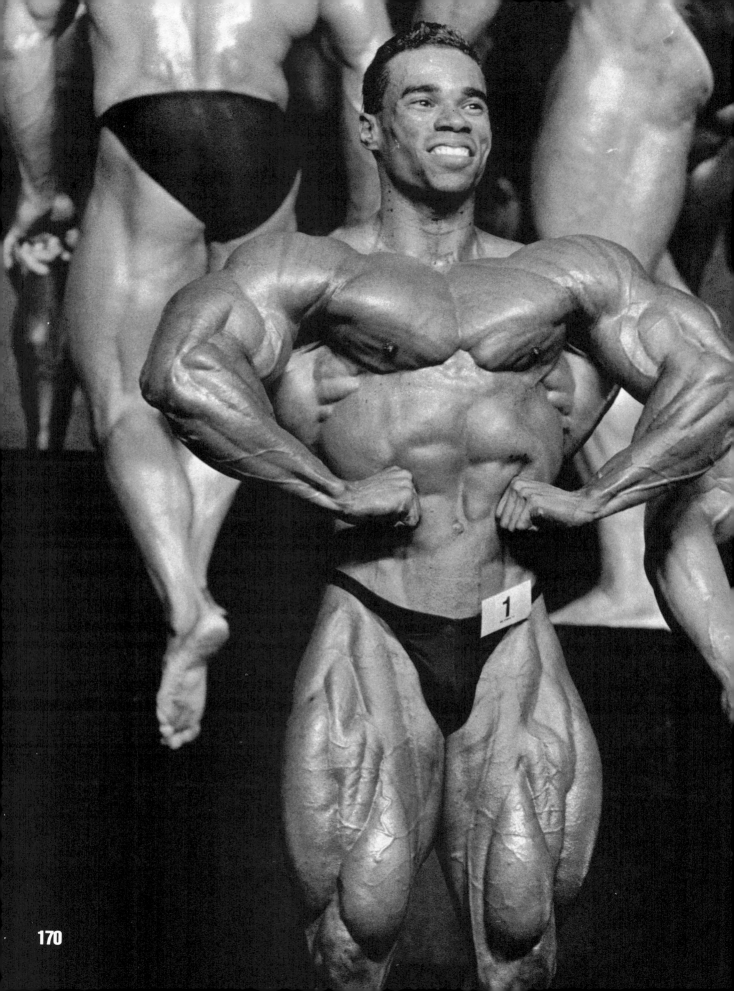

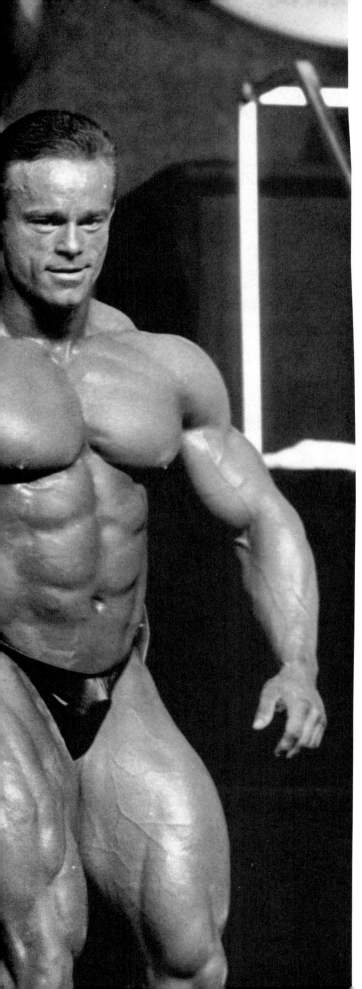

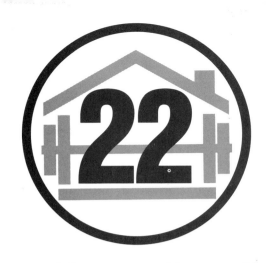

In exercising your quadriceps and hamstrings with barbells, you're going to work your gluteals as well. But this is to your advantage. The gluteals are perhaps the thickest muscles in your body, and when well developed, they add a powerful look to your physique.

Strong, shapely, and separated quadriceps and hamstrings are not easy to build. They take concentrated exercise and a desire on your part to push through the pain barrier. As Arthur Jones said once, "Working your thighs properly should make you feel as though you have just climbed a tall building with your car tied to your back."

Get ready to climb a tall building with the following double pre-exhaustion cycle.

DOUBLE PRE-EXHAUSTION
THIGH CYCLE

Double pre-exhaustion stacks three related exercises back-to-back. Be sure to have everything arranged beforehand, because as little as three seconds' rest between the exercises will reduce the effectiveness of the cycle.

Kevin Levrone was awarded second place in his first Mr. Olympia. His thighs are outstanding.

1. Half squat with barbell:

Load the barbell with at least fifty more pounds than you normally squat with for ten repetitions. Instead of going down with the weight until the backs of your thighs come in full contact with your calves, descend only halfway or until your back thighs are approximately parallel with the floor. Do eight to twelve half squats with as much weight as you can handle. After the final repetition, move quickly into position for the sissy squat.

2. Sissy squat :

Initially, use only your body weight as a source of resistance. Lean back and bend only your knees as you lower and raise your body smoothly. Your thighs should be on fire with pain as you do the last repetition. With your partner's help, immediately get back to the squat racks.

The first two exercises have effectively pre-exhausted the fronts of your thighs. Your hamstrings and gluteals are now called into action on the regular squat to force your fatigued quadriceps to a deeper level of growth stimulation. One tip: use significantly less resistance on the squat than you use normally.

3. Squat with barbell:

You won't feel like doing deep squats immediately after the half squat and sissy squat, but you must for the dramatic results you're after. Take a deep breath and lower your body slowly to the bottom position. Return to the standing position. Repeat for maximum repetitions.

SALIENT ADVICE

The double pre-exhaustion thigh cycle takes less than five minutes to perform, but that five minutes will be like no other five minutes you've ever experienced. You may have a tendency to become nauseous afterward on your first workout. If so, take it easy at first. This feeling should disappear after your initial training session.

To the thigh cycle, I recommend that you add the following exercises to round out your routine:

1. Half squat with barbell, immediately followed by
2. Sissy squat, immediately followed by
3. Squat with barbell

---

4. Straight-armed pullover with one dumbbell
5. Shoulder shrug with barbell
6. Press behind neck with barbell
7. Bend-over row with barbell
8. Bench press with barbell
9. Biceps curl with barbell
10. Triceps extension with one dumbbell
11. Chin-up
12. Dip

This routine is composed of three exercises for your lower body and nine for your upper body. Do the complete routine twice a week, on Monday and on Friday. On Wednesday, do only the nine upper-body exercises.

Twice-a-week thigh training produces the best growth stimulation in almost all cases. This pre-exhaustion thigh cycle, however, should not be done more than twice a week for four consecutive weeks. Doing more would simply be too demanding on your

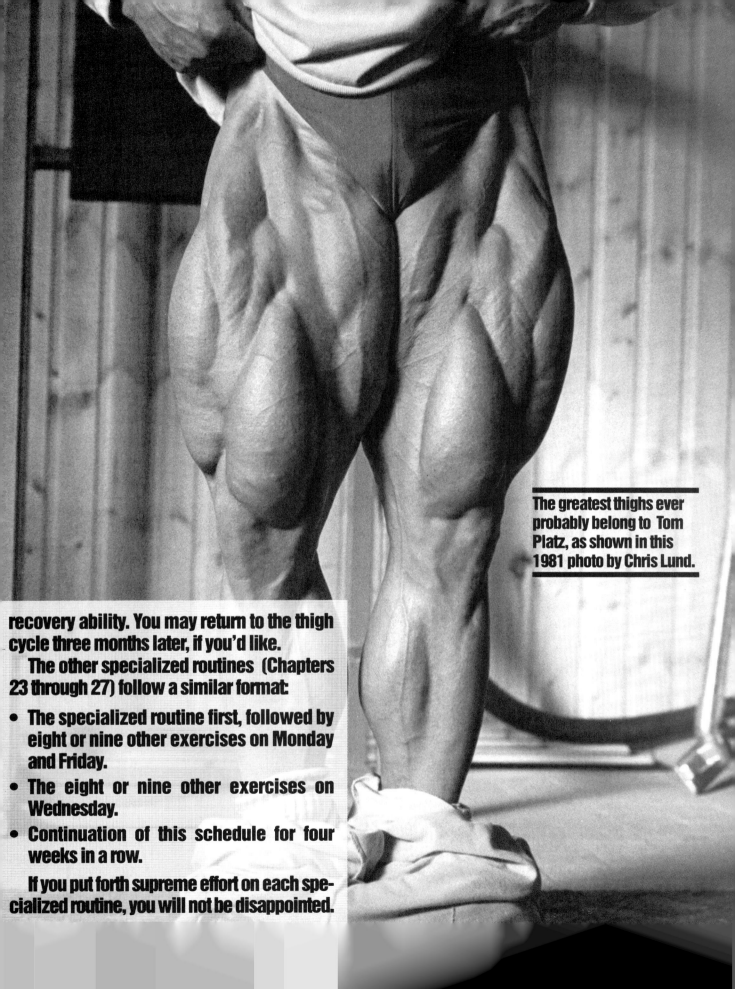

The greatest thighs ever probably belong to Tom Platz, as shown in this 1981 photo by Chris Lund.

recovery ability. You may return to the thigh cycle three months later, if you'd like.

The other specialized routines (Chapters 23 through 27) follow a similar format:

- The specialized routine first, followed by eight or nine other exercises on Monday and Friday.
- The eight or nine other exercises on Wednesday.
- Continuation of this schedule for four weeks in a row.

If you put forth supreme effort on each specialized routine, you will not be disappointed.

CHAPTER 23
CALVES: FULL AND FLARED

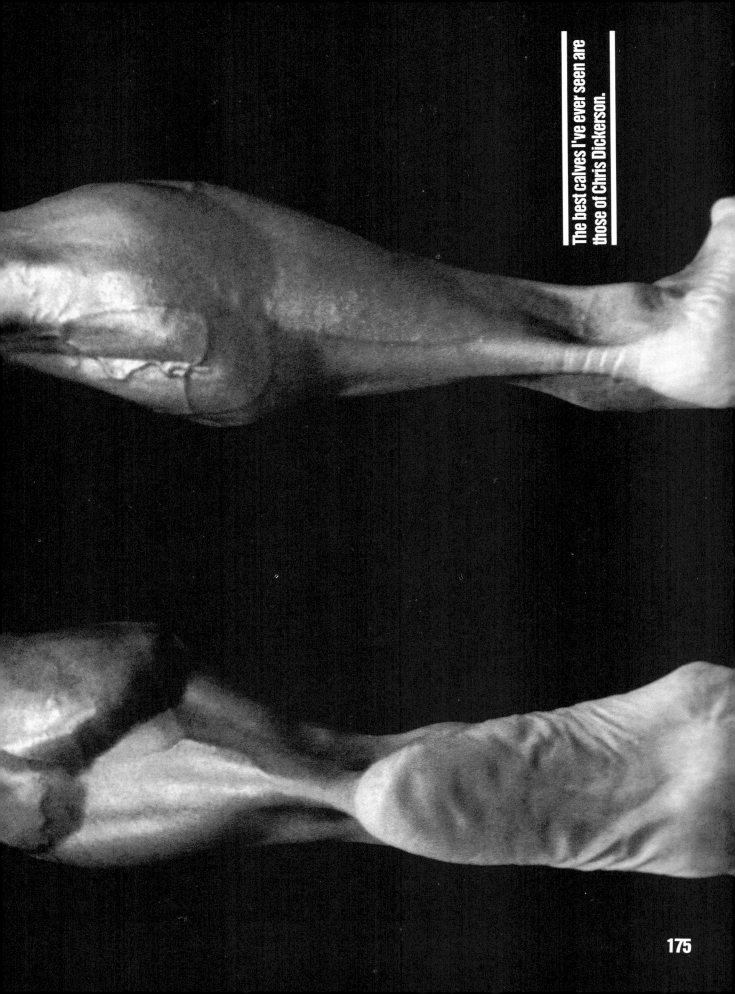

The best calves I've ever seen are those of Chris Dickerson.

175

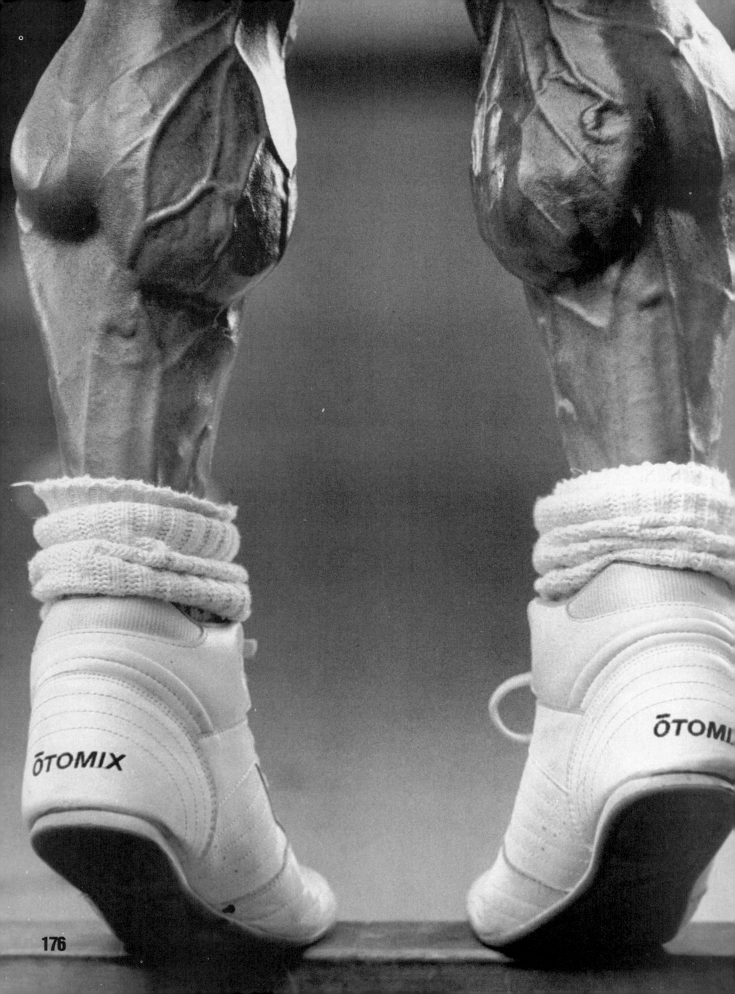

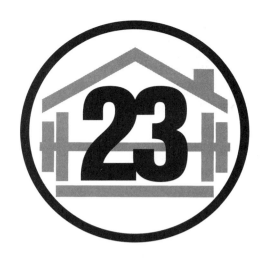

I've seen some great calves in my more than thirty years of interest in bodybuilding. For example, I remember well the calves of Steve Reeves and Mike Mentzer. More recently, the lower legs of Paul DeMayo and Mike Matarazzo are outstanding in all aspects.

However, the calves that remain etched in my mind as the best ever—the fullest, most flared, the deepest cut—are those of Chris Dickerson. Dickerson won the 1970 Mr. America and the 1982 Mr. Olympia.

There's an interesting fact that not many people know about Chris Dickerson. As great as his calves are, he has a twin brother who has even better lower legs. And here's the interesting sidebar: Chris's brother has never done any bodybuilding; he has never tried to develop his calves. This leads me to believe that if Chris had avoided training his calves, they may have been even bigger. Perhaps Chris's calves might be smaller than their full potential because of overtraining.

You should also understand that Chris and his brother have extremely long gastroc-soleus muscles, which is why their calves

The calves of Paul DeMayo are attention-getters.

are so wide and diamond-shaped. Only a little exercise works wonders on such unusual muscle bellies.

The rest of us who aren't so gifted in the calf department need a well-organized plan to build our lower legs. But that well-organized plan must become briefer as it becomes harder.

Here is a calf routine that will get your attention.

PRE-EXHAUSTION CALF CYCLE

1. One-legged calf raise with dumbbell:

A sturdy four-inch block of wood is necessary to perform this exercise. In a standing position with the dumbbell in your left hand, place the ball of your left foot on the block. Use your right arm to hold on to something to stabilize your body. While keeping your left knee locked, raise and lower your heel in a smooth, slow manner. Concentrate on contracting at the top and stretching at the bottom. When your left calf is exhausted, switch the dumbbell to your right hand and repeat the procedure for your right calf. After you've worked your right calf, walk around for thirty seconds or so before the next exercise. You do not have to rush.

2. Seated calf raise:

This movement works your soleus, a large flat muscle that lies beneath your gastrocnemius. Well-developed soleus muscles add dramatic fullness and flare to your lower legs. The seated calf raise is an exercise that requires a few trials to master. Sit in front of the block of wood and place the balls of your feet on the wood. Your knees are bent at approximately ninety degrees. A pillow goes on your knees, and a board that's wide enough for your partner to sit on goes across the pillow. Your partner now sits on the board and you're ready to begin lifting and lowering your heels. Lift your heels smoothly and try to extend on your big toes. Pause. Lower slowly and repeat for maximum repetitions. After the last repetition, immediately move to the donkey calf raise.

3. Donkey calf raise:

With your partner across your hips, perform eight to twelve slow repetitions. Remember to take a full four seconds up and four seconds down on each repetition. And keep your knees locked. At the end of this exercise your calves should feel like footballs.

THE REST OF THE ROUTINE

Here's the recommended routine to follow for the next month:

1. One-legged calf raise with dumbbell
2. Seated calf raise, immediately followed by
3. Donkey calf raise

---

4. Bent-armed pullover with barbell
5. Upright row with barbell
6. Incline press with barbell
7. Bent-over raise with dumbbells
8. Decline press with barbell
9. Bent-over row with barbell
10. Reverse curl with barbell
11. Trunk curl
12. Stiff-legged deadlift with barbell or squat with barbell

As with the thighs (Chapter 22), the calf

cycle and the other nine exercises are done on Mondays and Fridays for four weeks. The other exercises, minus the calf cycle, are performed on Wednesdays.

Exercise 12, the stiff-legged deadlift or the squat, merits some explanation. They should be alternated. On Monday and Friday of one week do the stiff-legged deadlift, and on Wednesday do the squat. The next week, do the squat on Monday and Friday and the stiff-legged deadlift on Wednesday. Continue with this same alternation for the other two weeks.

Your calves can improve dramatically in only four weeks. Keep your form strict. Make each repetition count. Look forward to the burn.

It was often said that Tom Platz's thighs overpowered the rest of his body. In this pose, however, his calves look overpowering.

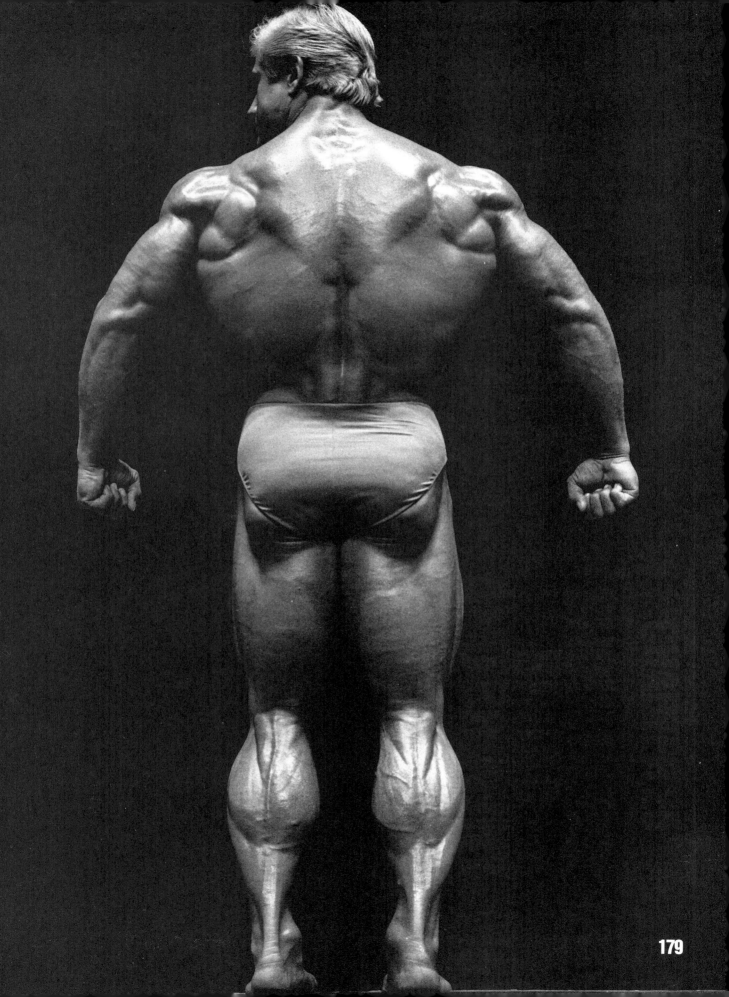

CHAPTER 24
BACK: WIDE AND DEEP

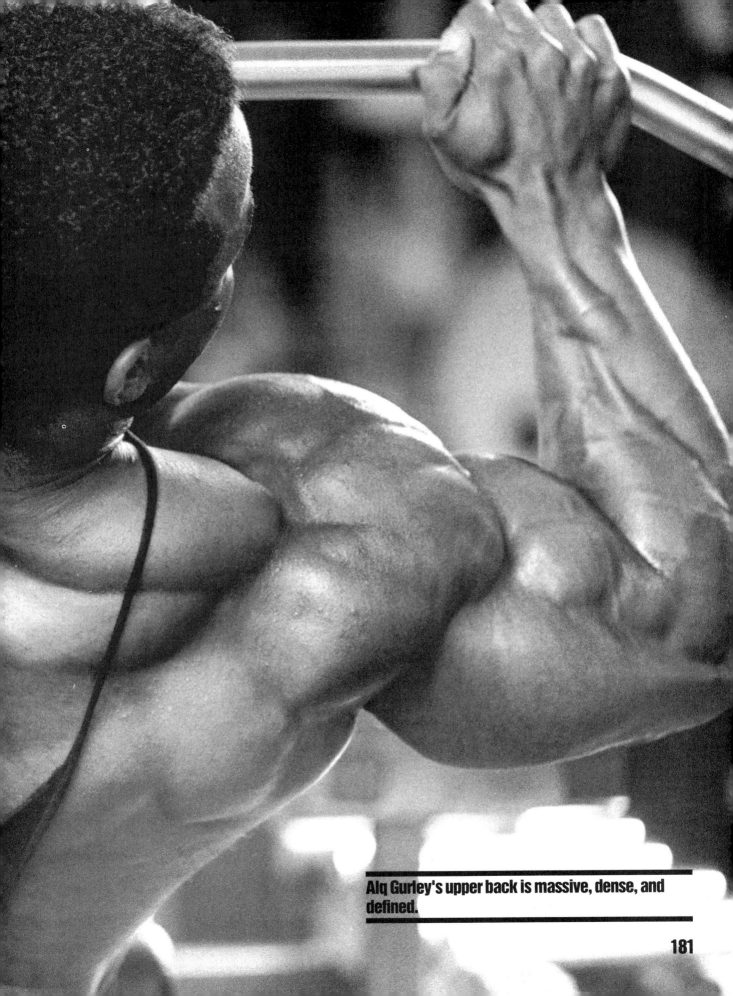

Alq Gurley's upper back is massive, dense, and defined.

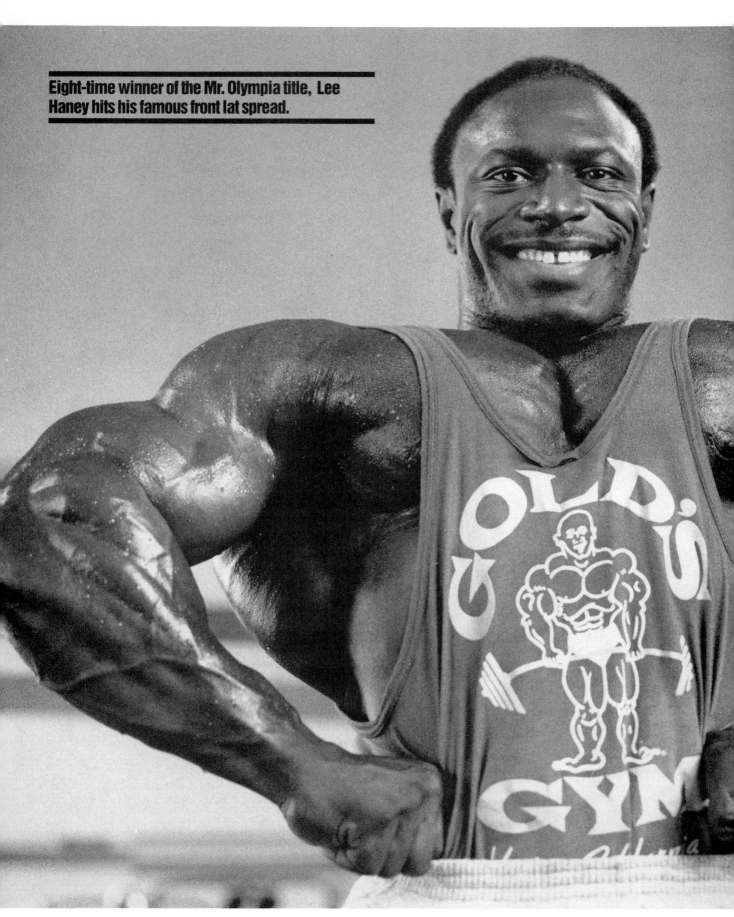

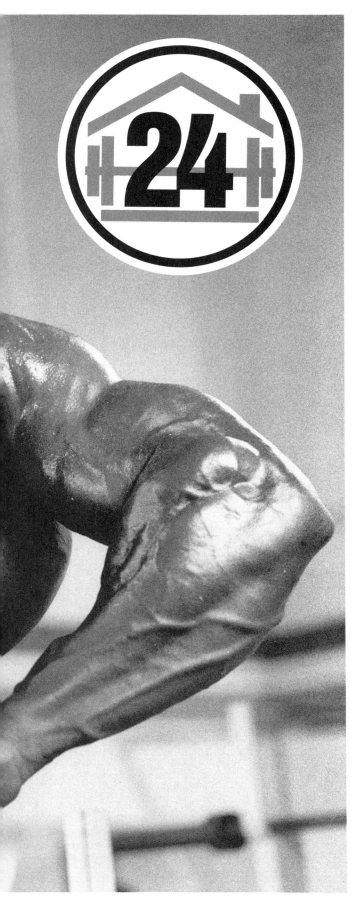

The best back in bodybuilding today still belongs to eight-time Mr. Olympia, Lee Haney. Haney's back is incredibly wide, especially in the lower lat area. But even more impressive than his width is his thickness. From his lumbar to the mid-back, up through his shoulder and neck region, Haney's mounds of muscle make him the deepest-muscled bodybuilder ever, at least when viewed from the back.

Granted Dorian Yates, as he appeared at the 1992 Mr. Olympia, is a close second. But Dorian's thickness is still not up to Haney's in his prime.

The back may take more time to develop than any other body part. Even with the correct genetic potential, it takes years (perhaps many) to get the championship width and depth. As with anything meaningful that takes time, the quest begins with a single step.

The following double pre-exhaustion cycle will put you several steps closer to your goal.

DOUBLE PRE-EXHAUSTION BACK CYCLE

1. Bent-over row with barbell:

With as much weight as you can handle, do eight to twelve repetitions in strict form. Instantly move to the bent-armed pullover.

2. Bent-armed pullover with barbell:

Move the barbell smoothly across your face and down and back for as many repetitions as possible. After the final repetition, place the barbell on the floor and run to the chinning bar.

3. Chin-up, negative-only:

Your lats are now exhausted. It's up to your

biceps to force the deeper muscle fibers of your lats to be called into action. Climb into the top position with your chin over the bar. Use a palms-up grip and space your hands shoulder-width apart. Remove your feet and lower your body very slowly to the bottom. This slow, negative work should take ten seconds at least on the first several repetitions. Your partner calls out the time and paces you during each negative-only repetition. Once at the bottom, quickly climb back to the top position and repeat. When you can no longer control your speed of lowering, stop. When you can do more than twelve repetitions in correct style, hang a twenty-five-pound weight or dumbbell to your waist with a belt or rope.

AFTER THE BACK CYCLE

When you complete the back cycle, you may take a brief rest period of several minutes. Then it's on to the remainder of your workout:

1. Bent-over row with barbell, immediately followed by
2. Bent-armed pullover with barbell, immediately followed by
3. Chin-up, negative-only

---

4. Leg curl machine
5. Leg extension machine
6. Donkey calf raise
7. Overhead press with barbell
8. Shoulder shrug with barbell
9. Bench press with barbell
10. Biceps curl with barbell
11. Triceps extension with one dumbbell
12. Reverse trunk curl

If the leg curl and leg extension machines are not at your disposal, substitute instead the stiff-legged deadlift and the sissy squat. Otherwise, perform each of the listed exercises as previously described for one set of eight to twelve repetitions. Regardless of the repetitions that you complete, always try one more. Remember, nothing takes the place of outright hard work!

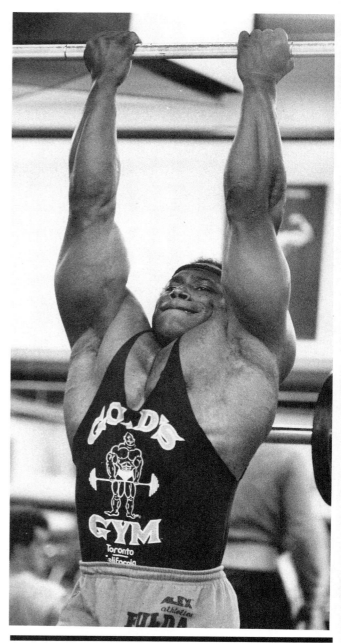

Chin-ups with a palms-up grip are one of the best exercises for your latissimus dorsi.

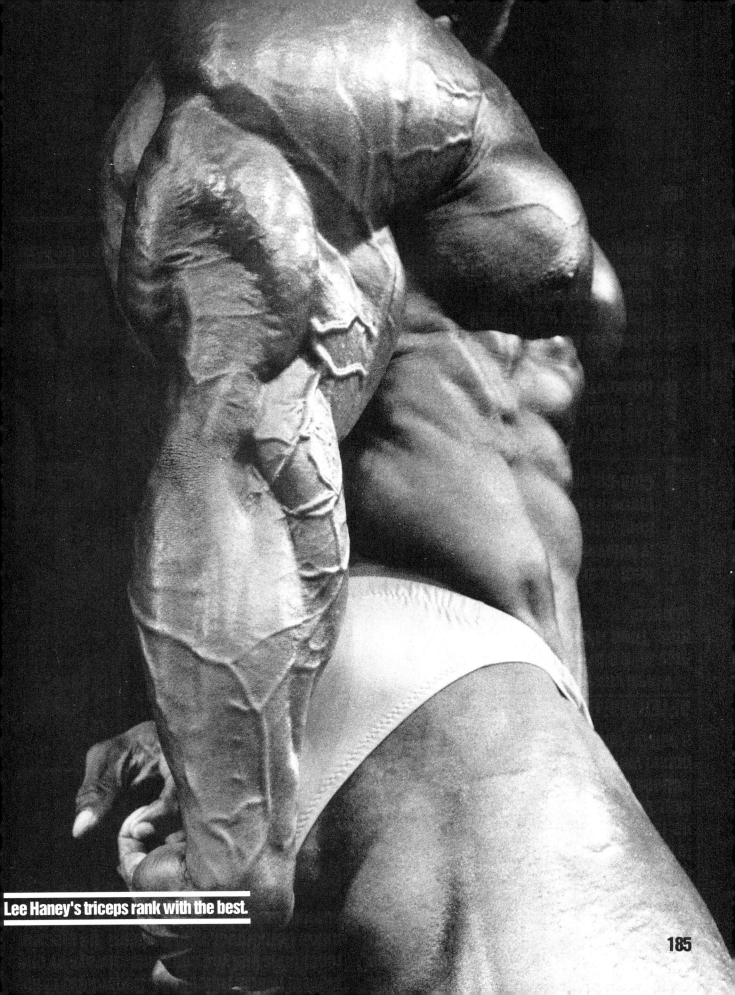

Lee Haney's triceps rank with the best.

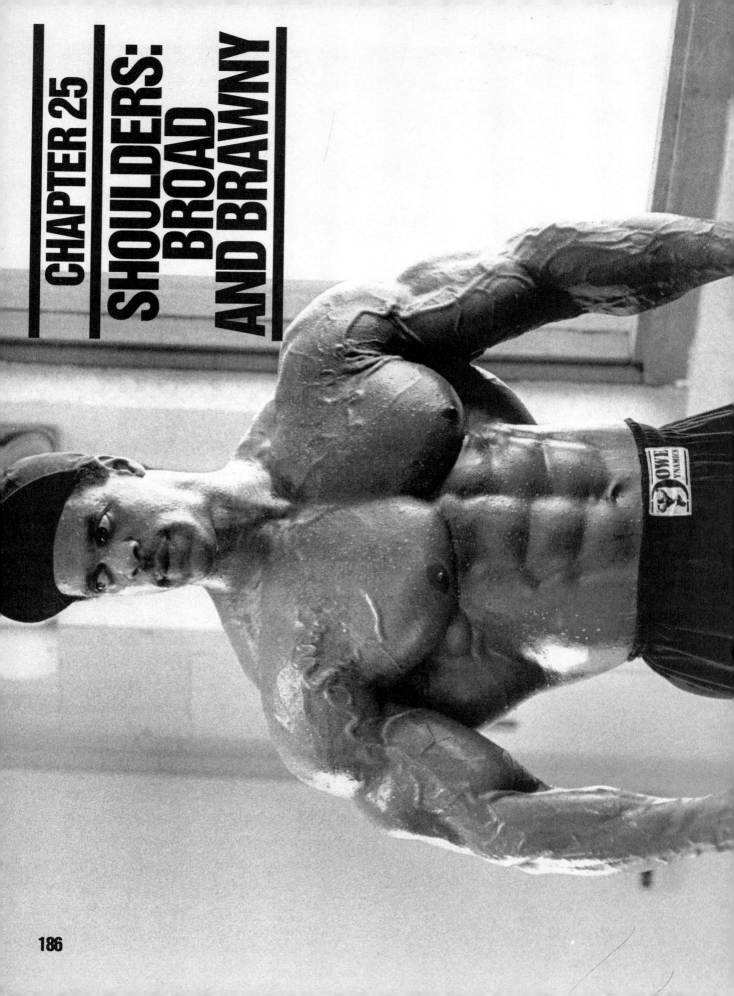

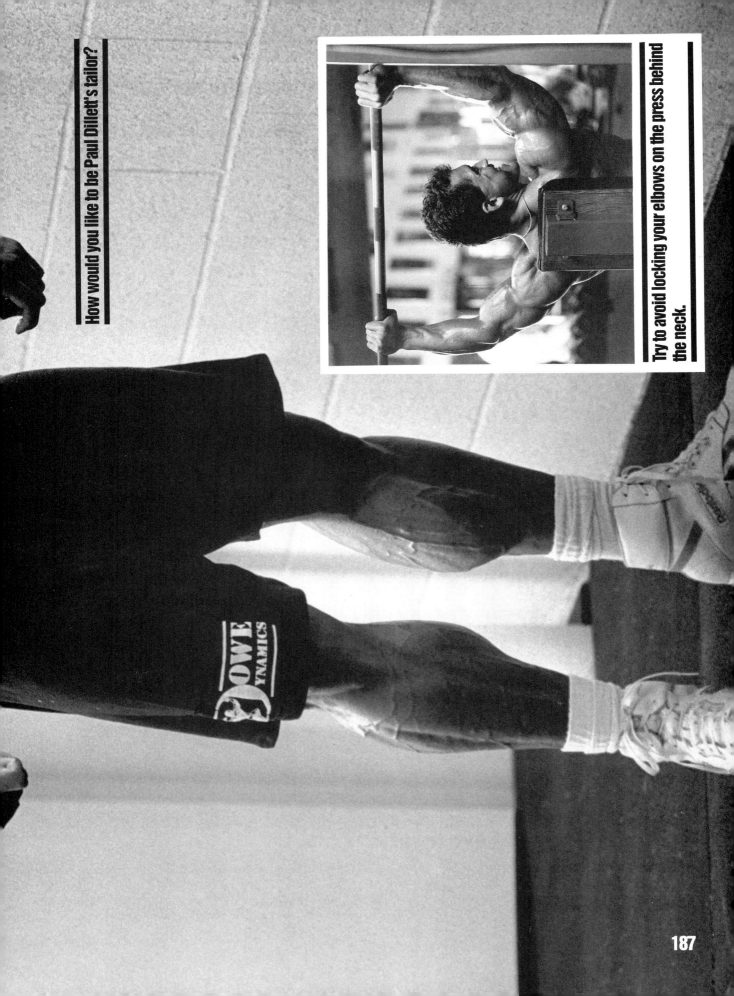

How would you like to be Paul Dillett's tailor?

Try to avoid locking your elbows on the press behind the neck.

187

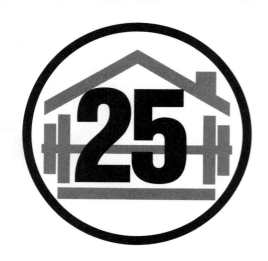

Nothing sets a bodybuilder off like massive shoulders. You can hide just about every part of your body. But you can't hide broad, brawny shoulders. Of course, who'd want to hide broad shoulders? Not you and not me!

Impressive shoulders are primarily the result of having strong, thick, and rounded deltoid muscles. Here's a double pre-exhaustion cycle that will blast your shoulders to new growth.

DOUBLE PRE-EXHAUSTION SHOULDER CYCLE

1. Overhead press with barbell:

You can make this exercise tougher by not locking out your elbows at the top. Lower the weight slowly and repeat for maximum repetitions. Replace the barbell on the floor and stand with a pair of dumbbells for the lateral raise.

2. Lateral raise with dumbbells:

Keep your elbows locked as you raise and lower the dumbbells to momentary muscular failure. You should be feeling this in your middle deltoids as you move to the press behind neck.

3. Press behind neck with barbell:

Place your hands a little wider apart than you do for the overhead press. Lift and lower the barbell smoothly behind your neck. Once again you can make this movement harder by not quite locking your elbows at the top. After five or six nonlocking repetitions, however, you can actually assist yourself by locking out. Locking out will provide you with a brief rest, which allows you to recover just enough to do several more repetitions.

THE NEW ROUTINE

After the shoulder cycle, you'll hit your legs, torso, and arms with these exercises:

1. Overhead press with barbell, immediately followed by
2. Lateral raise with dumbbells, immediately followed by
3. Press behind neck

---

4. Squat with barbell or stiff-legged deadlift with barbell
5. Straight-armed pullover with one dumbbell
6. Bent-armed fly with dumbbells
7. Chin-up
8. Dip
9. Biceps curl with dumbbells
10. Triceps kickback with dumbbells
11. Wrist curl with barbell
12. Trunk curl

Give this routine your best effort over the next four weeks and you'll be well on your way to having broad and brawny shoulders.

Dumbbells allow you a lot of variety in working your shoulders.

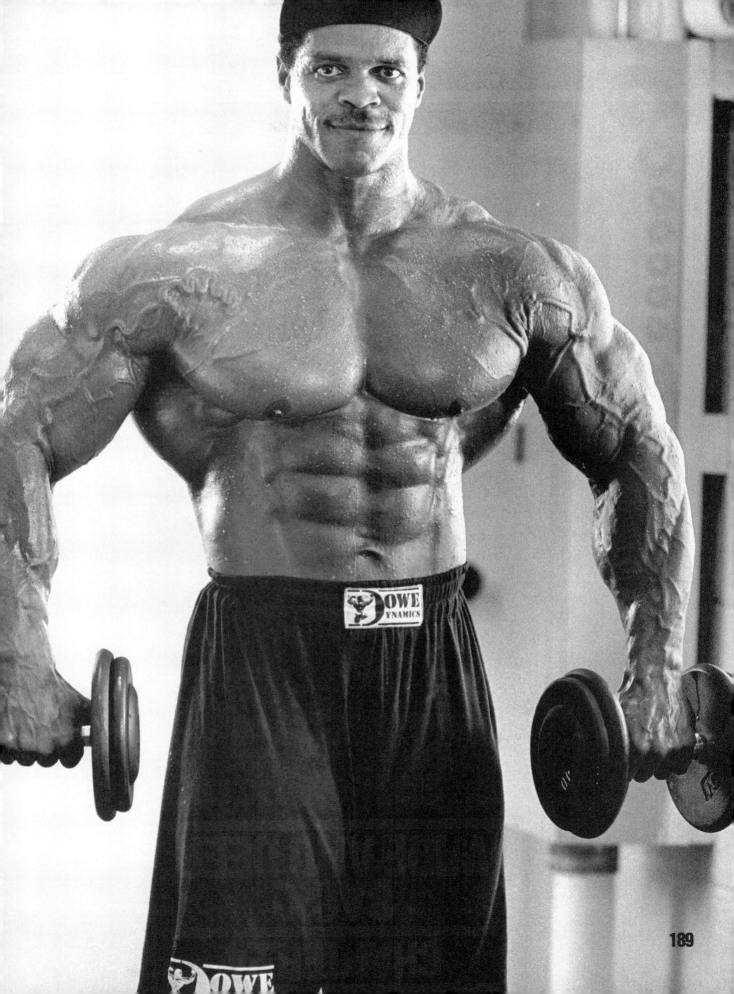

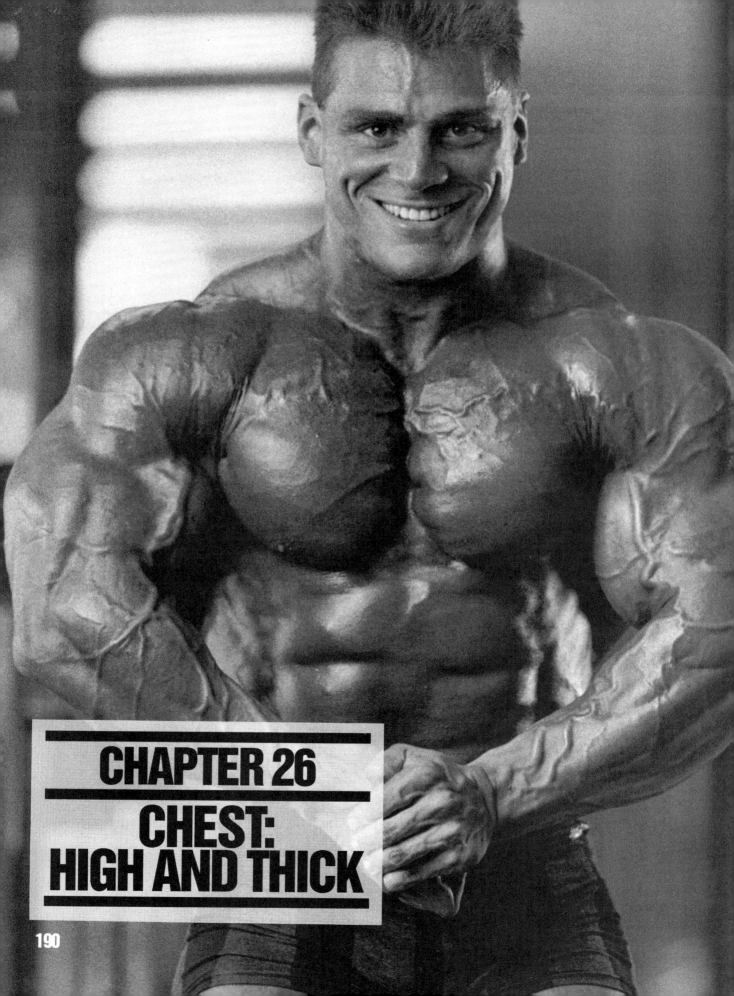

CHAPTER 26
CHEST: HIGH AND THICK

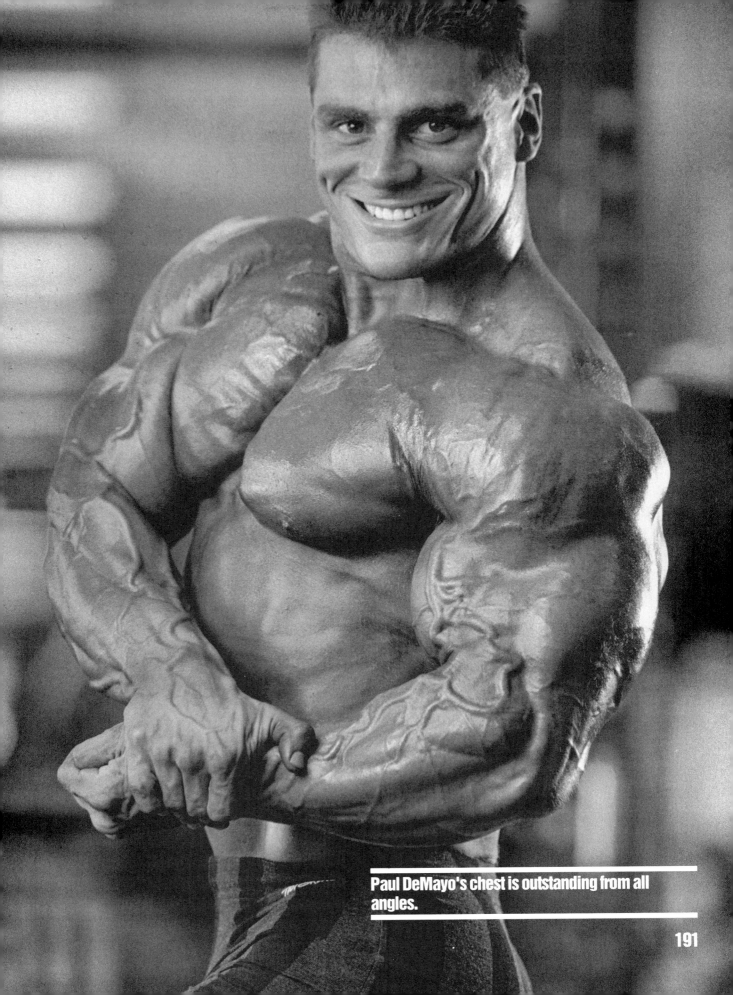

Paul DeMayo's chest is outstanding from all angles.

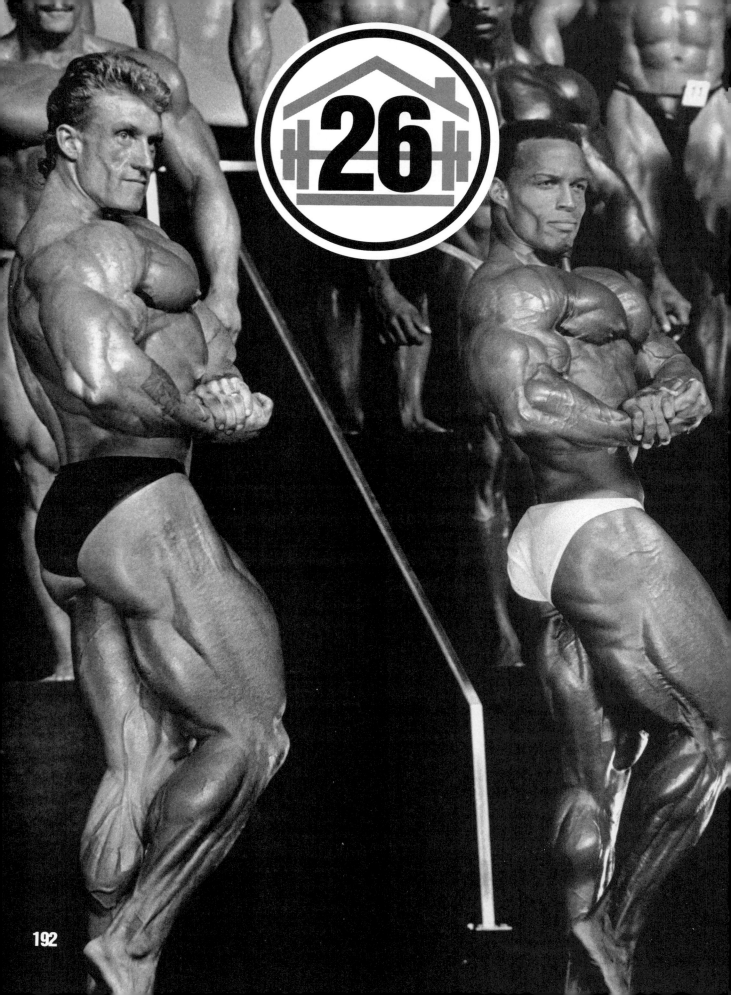

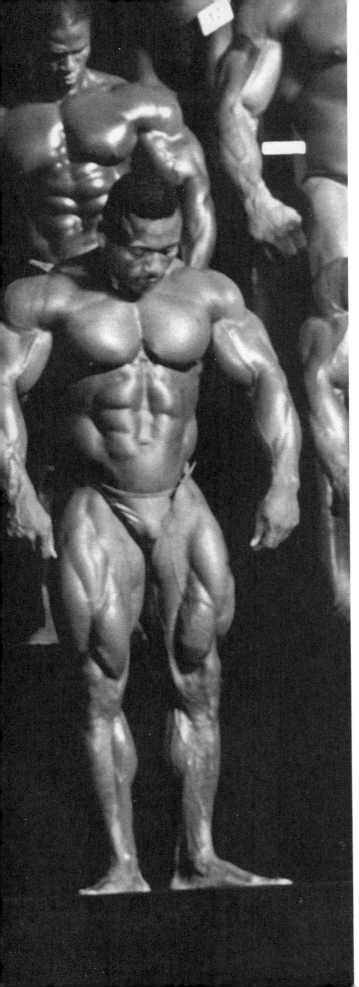

Many muscles surround the chest area, but the most important is the pectoralis major. It has a broad origin along the sternum and the clavicle. It then fans across the chest and inserts on the front of the upper arm bone.

When the pectoral muscles contract, they pull the upper arms across the body. Doing so involves the lower and middle muscle fibers. To develop the much-desired upper fibers for that high-chest look, the arms must be angled at an incline in relation to the torso.

Thus, for full chest development, you need an exercise for the middle and lower pectorals, as well as one for the upper region. That's exactly what this double pre-exhaustion cycle supplies.

DOUBLE PRE-EXHAUSTION
CHEST CYCLE

1. Incline press with barbell:

An incline bench of forty-five degrees is best for this exercise. Position your hands on the bar slightly wider than your shoulders. Lift the barbell over your upper chest. Lower the bar slowly while keeping your elbows wide. Touch your chest and press the bar back until your arms are almost straight. Repeat for eight to twelve repetitions. After the last repetition, get ready for the bent-armed fly.

2. Bent-armed fly with dumbbells:

Reposition your body on a flat bench with a dumbbell in either hand. Do the bent-armed fly for as many repetitions as possible. You should definitely feel this in your pectorals. Immediately move to the dip bars.

Dorian Yates and Shawn Ray compare chest poses.

3. Dip:

Mount the bar and start doing a smooth set of dips. If you can't perform at least eight repetitions, have your partner grasp your feet from behind and assist you by lifting up on your legs.

THE REST OF THE ROUTINE

1. Incline press with barbell, immediately followed by
2. Bent-armed fly with dumbbells, immediately followed by
3. Dip

---

4. Leg extension machine
5. Leg curl machine
6. Donkey calf raise
7. Upright row with barbell
8. Behind neck chin-up
9. Wrist curl with barbell
10. Reverse wrist curl with barbell
11. Reverse curl with barbell
12. Shoulder shrug with barbell

As in previous routines, perform the chest cycle on Mondays and Fridays along with the other nine exercises listed. On Wednesdays, do the last nine exercises only.

Your chest will expand quickly if the exercise is intense and progressive. Be positive and believe.

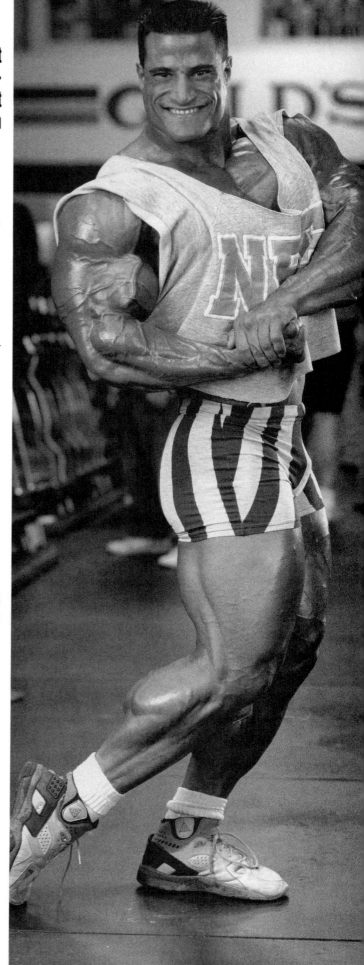

Take your shirt off, Mike. Show us your chest!

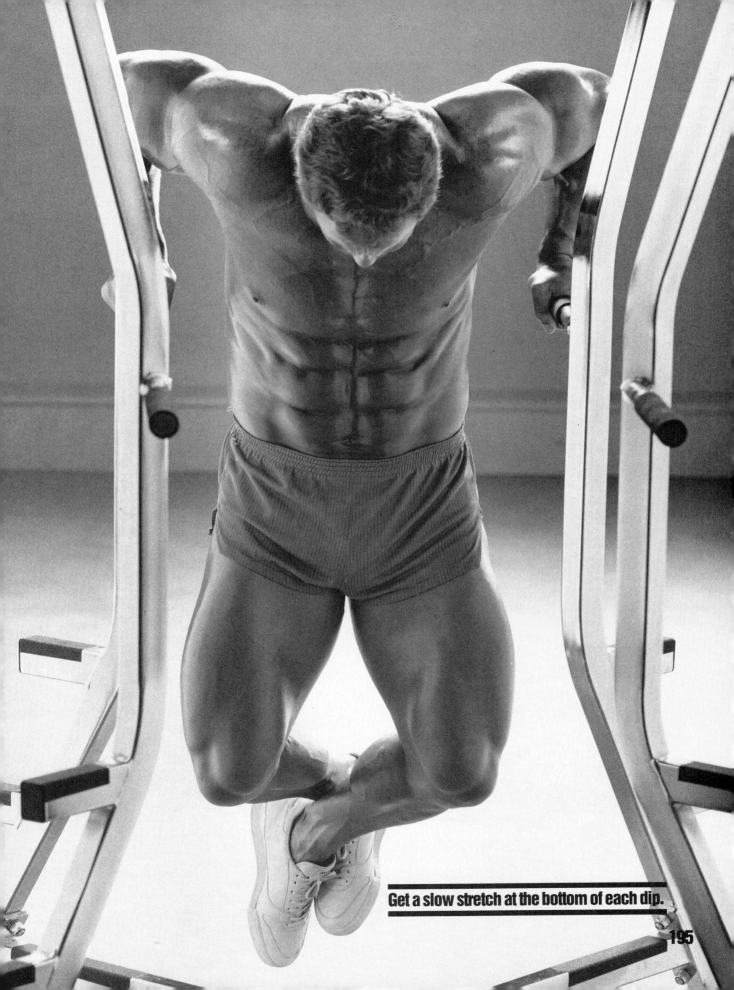

Get a slow stretch at the bottom of each dip.

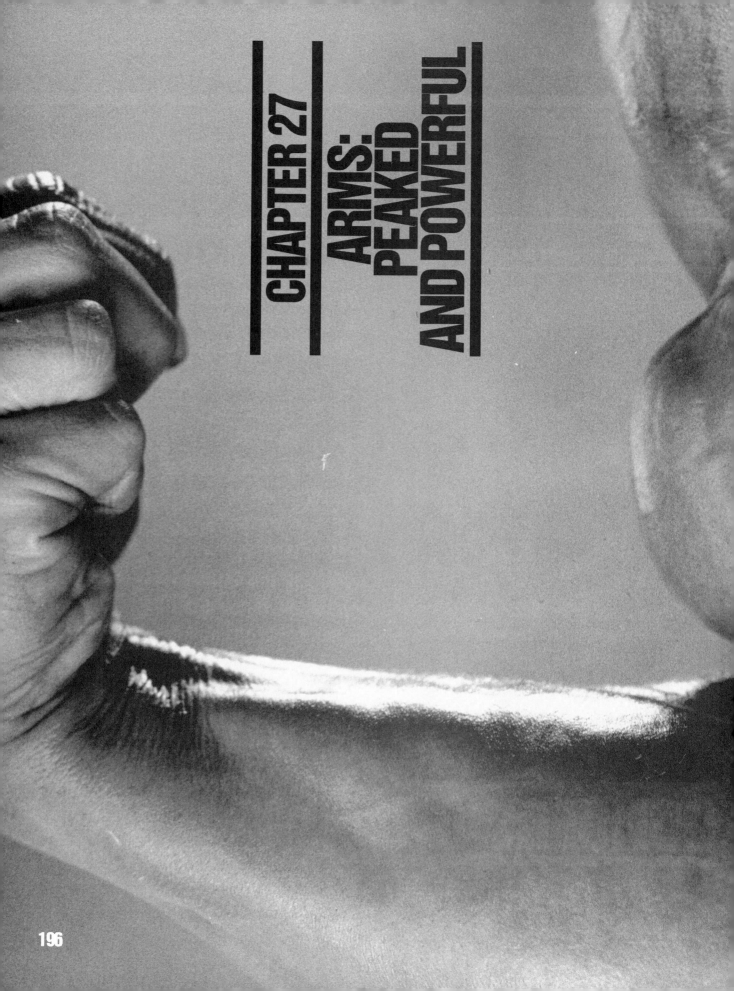

CHAPTER 27
ARMS: PEAKED AND POWERFUL

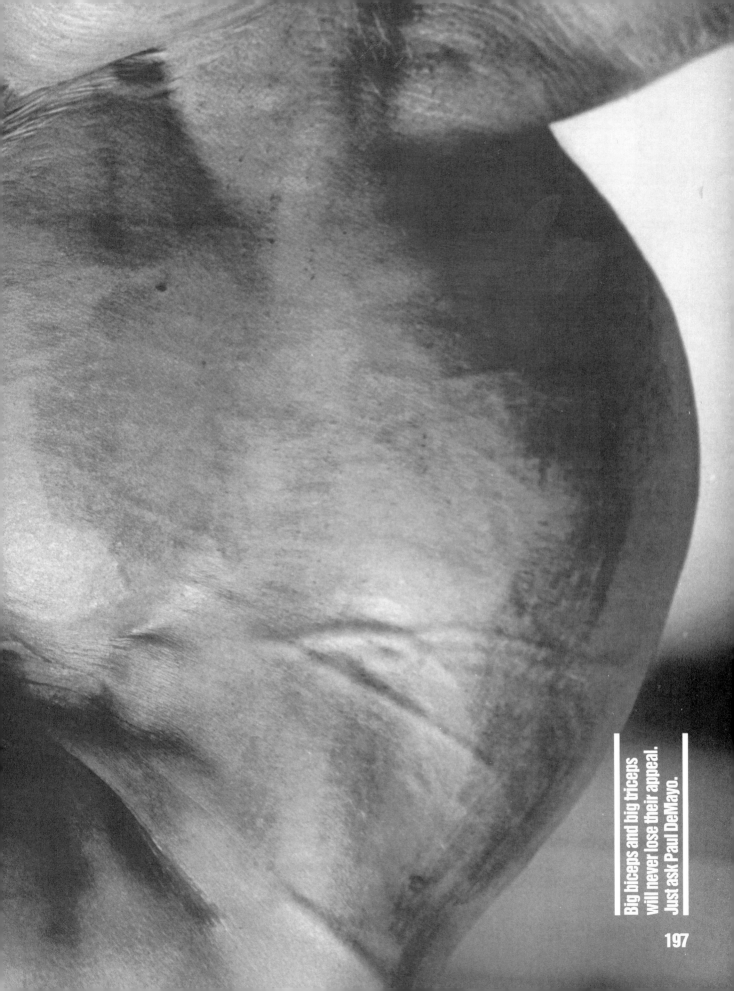

Big biceps and big triceps will never lose their appeal. Just ask Paul DeMayo.

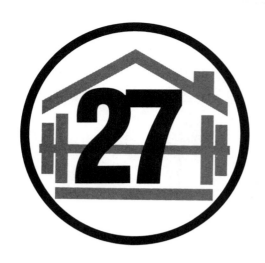

Biceps and triceps. Big arms. Unquestionably, the number-one topic in the bodybuilding world. Just how popular are arm-building articles in the muscle magazines?

Joe Roark, a muscle historian who writes a monthly column for <u>Flex</u>, reviewed every issue of nine different bodybuilding magazines over a ten-year time period. In all, he recorded 1,129 training articles from 573 magazines. Here's what he found:

There were 318 arm-building articles. In second place was back training, with 157 entries. Arm building was over twice as popular as back training.

Why is there so much interest in big arms? Probably because most trainees get nothing close to the results they are seeking from the workouts they are doing. Most of them, through misleading training articles, overwork their biceps and triceps.

Once again, the secret to peaked and powerful arms is hard, brief, infrequent exercise. Here are simple pre-exhaustion cycles—two exercises for your biceps and two exercises for your triceps—that fulfill all the essentials for efficient arm building.

PRE-EXHAUSTION ARM CYCLES

1. Biceps curl with barbell:

Do as many smooth, slow curls as you can. Make your biceps really ache to the bone. Instantly, run to the chinning bar.

2. Chin-up, negative-only:

Unlike the chin-up in the back cycle, your lats are not pre-exhausted. It's your biceps that are fatigued. Thus, you must use the fresh strength of your lats to force your pre-exhausted biceps to a deeper level of muscle-fiber involvement. Try to get at least eight slow, negative-only repetitions. Have your partner pace you closely in the downward phase. Keep your face relaxed as much as you can. You'll need to add weight to your body after you can perform twelve or more repetitions.

3. Triceps extension with one dumbbell:

This exercise zeros in on the long head of your triceps, which makes your arm look huge when it's hanging. Over the last several months, your triceps strength should be steadily on the rise. Put it to good use by progressing to a heavier dumbbell. Do eight to twelve strict repetitions of the triceps extension. Place the dumbbell on the floor and get to the dipping bars.

4. Dip, negative-only:

If you haven't tried hanging a twenty-five-pound dumbbell around your waist on this exercise, do so. Your triceps will thrive on the greater intensity. Again, have your partner pace you as you descend on each repetition. It really helps to keep your face relaxed, so concentrate on it. Always try to do one more repetition—under control, of course.

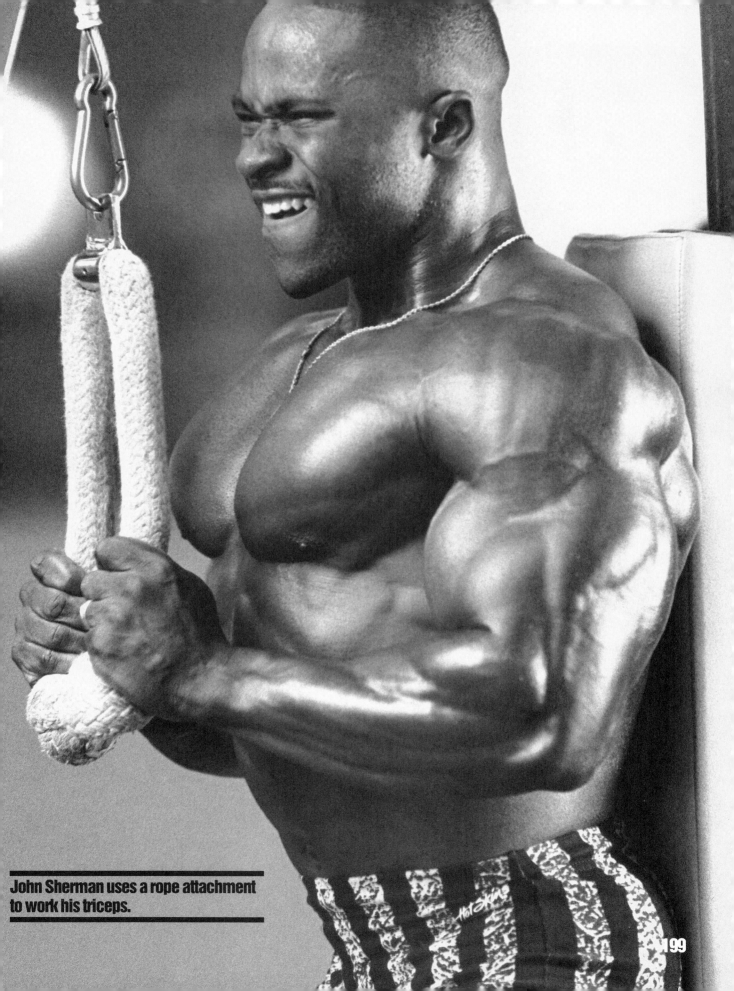

John Sherman uses a rope attachment to work his triceps.

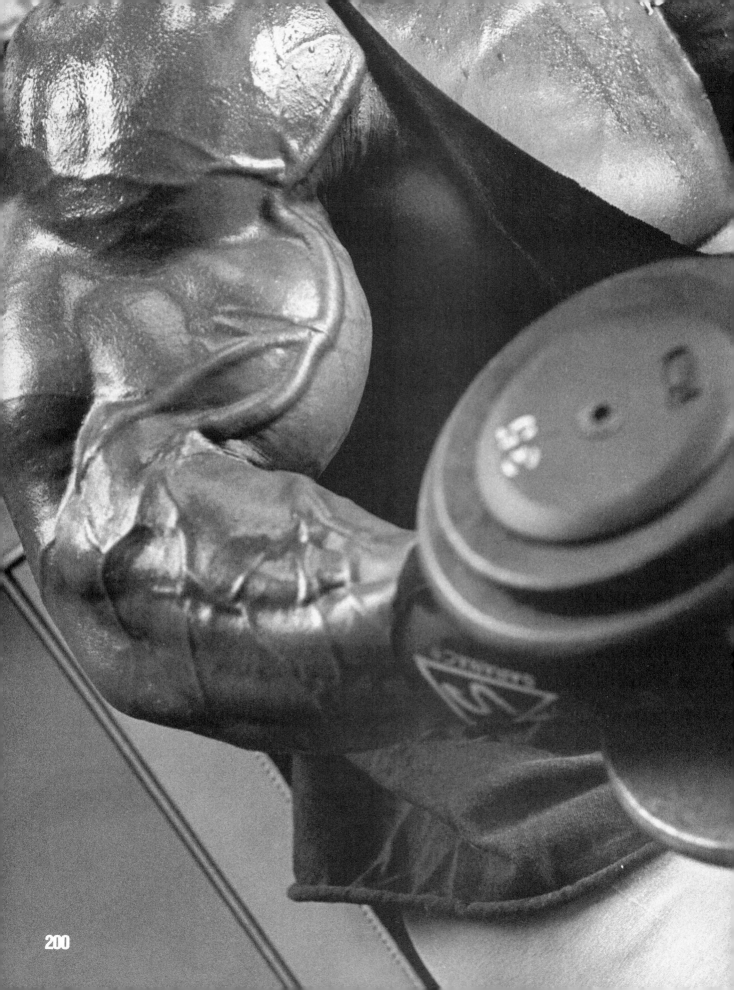

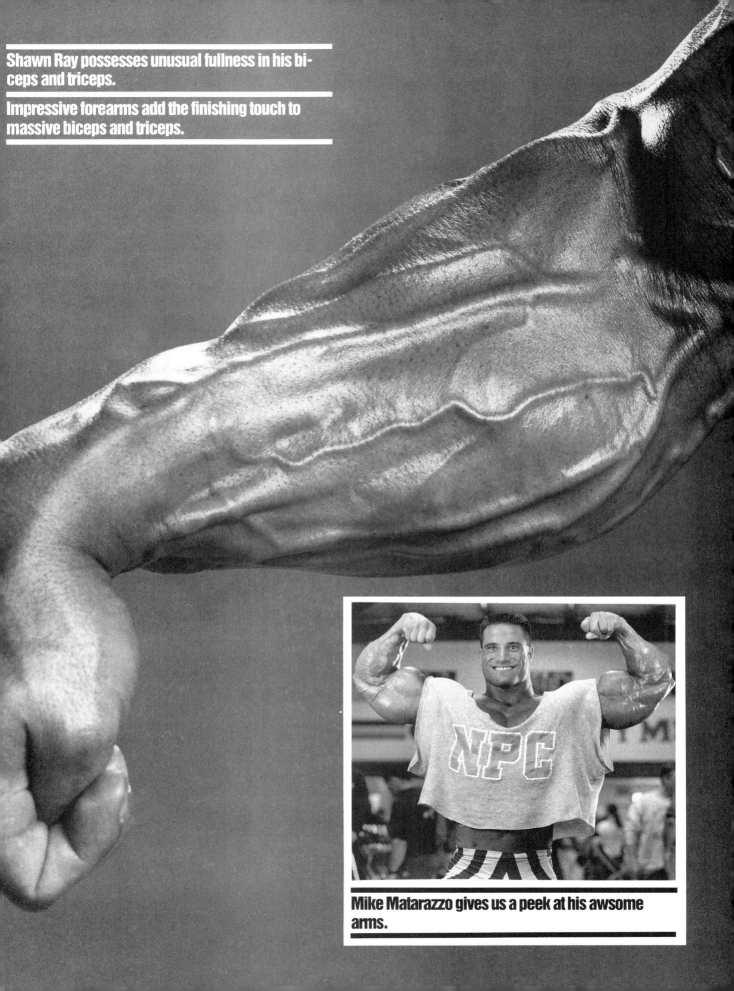

Shawn Ray possesses unusual fullness in his biceps and triceps.

Impressive forearms add the finishing touch to massive biceps and triceps.

Mike Matarazzo gives us a peek at his awsome arms.

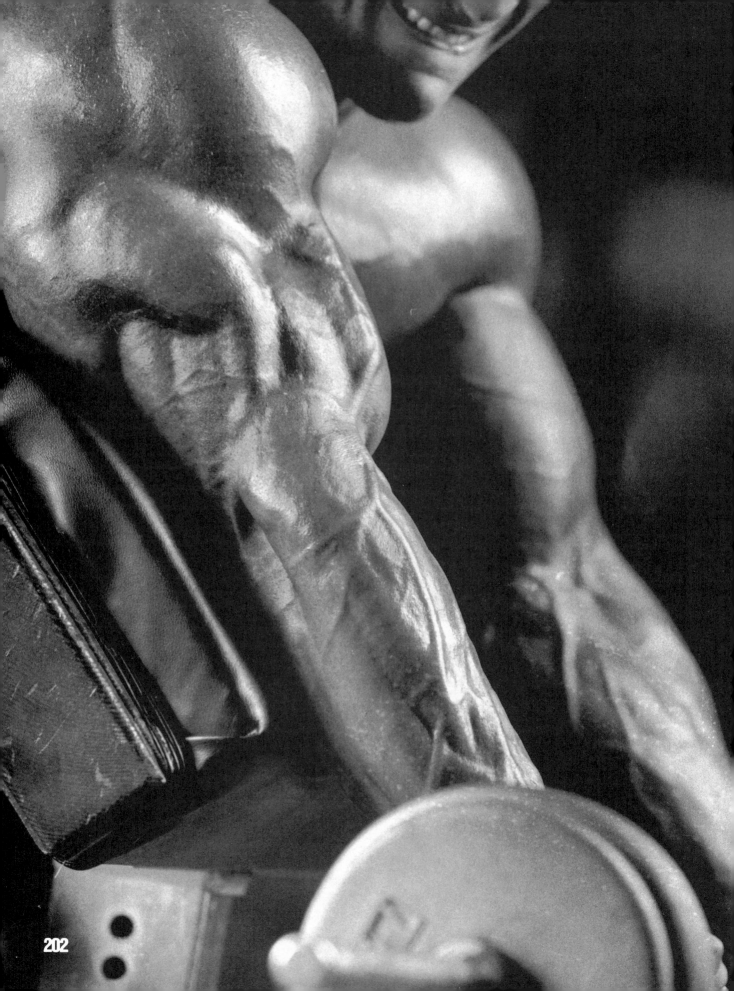

AFTER THE ARM CYCLES

1. Biceps curl with barbell, immediately followed by
2. Chin-up, negative-only
3. Triceps extension with one dumbbell, immediately followed by
4. Dip, negative-only

---

5. Squat with barbell or deadlift with barbell
6. Straight-armed pullover with one dumbbell
7. Seated calf raise
8. Bench press with barbell
9. Bent-over row with barbell
10. Lateral raise with dumbbells
11. Trunk curl
12. Reverse trunk curl

Be sure to perform the squat or the deadlift on an alternating basis. Do not practice both of them during the same workout.

Your workouts should now be honed to the point that they take no longer than thirty minutes to perform. Do not make the mistake of resting longer than a minute between most exercises. Furthermore, do not make the mistake of alternating with your partner on an exercise-by-exercise basis. Let him push you through the entire routine first. After a moderate rest period, you then push him through a similar workout.

Biceps and triceps. Big arms. If that's one of your goals, this arm cycle—which emphasizes negative work—will move you in a positive direction.

Curls on a preacher bench can help to stabilize your shoulders and elbows.

A FINAL NOTE:
PERSIST AND CONQUER!

The twenty-seven chapters in this manual provide you with the guts of getting through your first year of home training. Following the recommended plan of action for a year will establish the solid foundation for your continued success.

As an advanced bodybuilder, you'll want to progress by referring to some of my previous books, such as 100 High-Intensity Ways to Improve Your Bodybuilding and BIG.

Read, understand, and apply. Along the way, you'll be challenged. Meet the challenges with intelligent action.

Workout after workout, Week after week, Month after month: PERSIST and CONQUER!

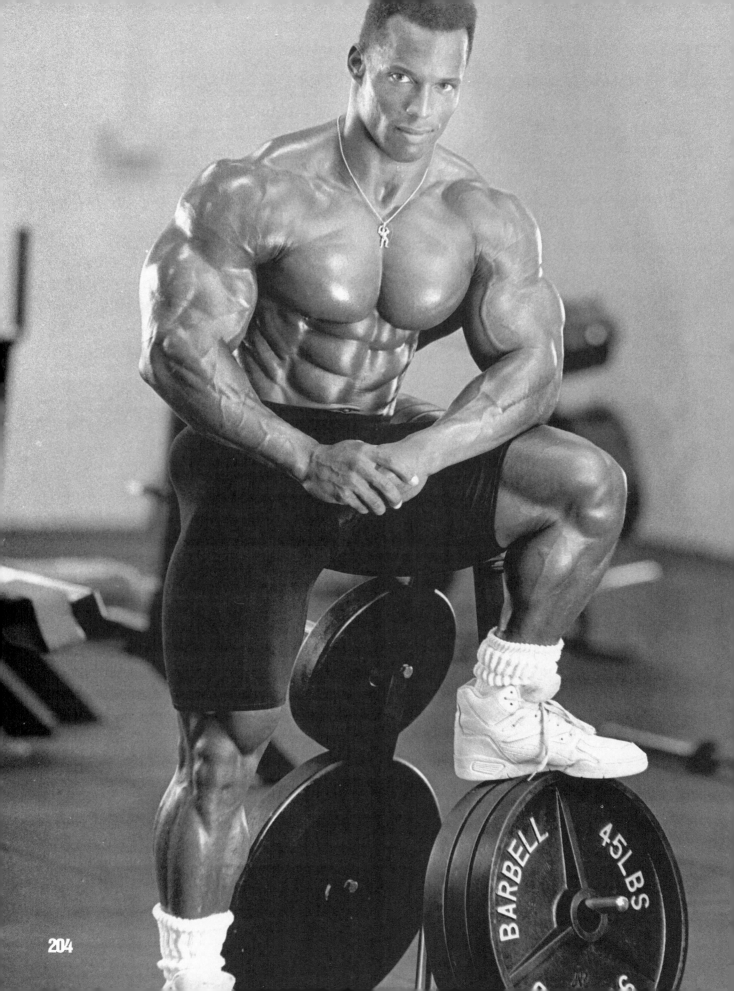

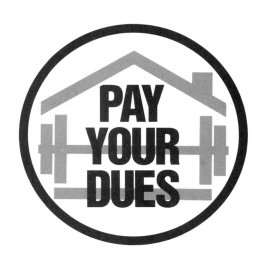

CONCLUSION

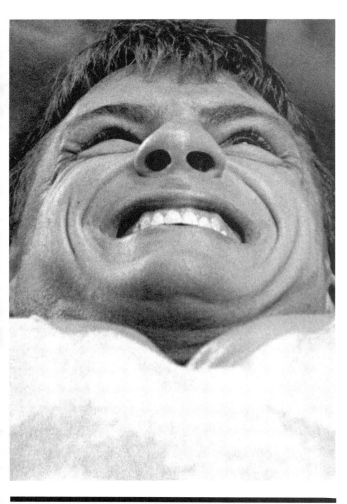

Understand and apply the rules of High-Intensity Home Training .

The goal of <u>High-Intensity Home Training</u> is to provide you with safe and efficient guidelines for building bigger and stronger muscles. The following is a summary of important rules:

- **Basic, not fancy**
- **Intensity, not duration**
- **Harder, not easier**
- **Repetitions, not lifts**
- **Smooth, not jerky**
- **Slow, not fast**
- **Briefer, not longer**
- **Infrequent, not daily**
- **Food, not supplements**
- **Rest, not drugs**
- **Quality, not quantity**
- **Results, not stagnation**

Impressive muscular development comes with a high price tag. The cost, however, can be overcome by the persistent application of the above guidelines.

DIG DEEP AND PAY YOUR DUES!

205

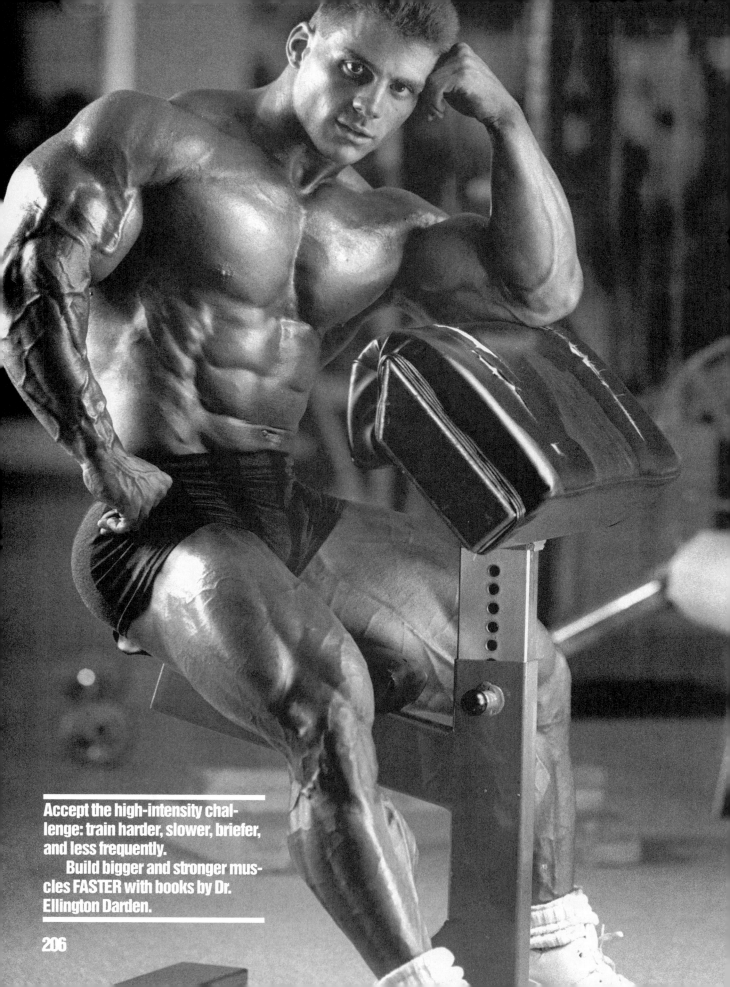

Accept the high-intensity challenge: train harder, slower, briefer, and less frequently.

Build bigger and stronger muscles FASTER with books by Dr. Ellington Darden.

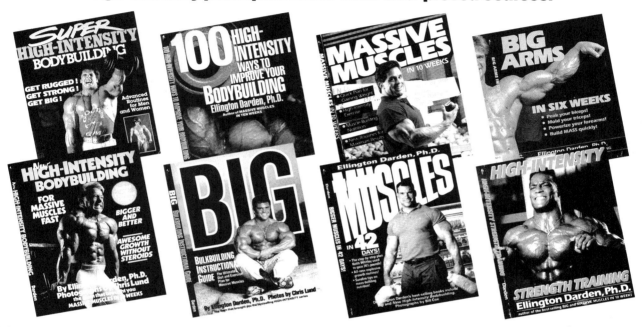

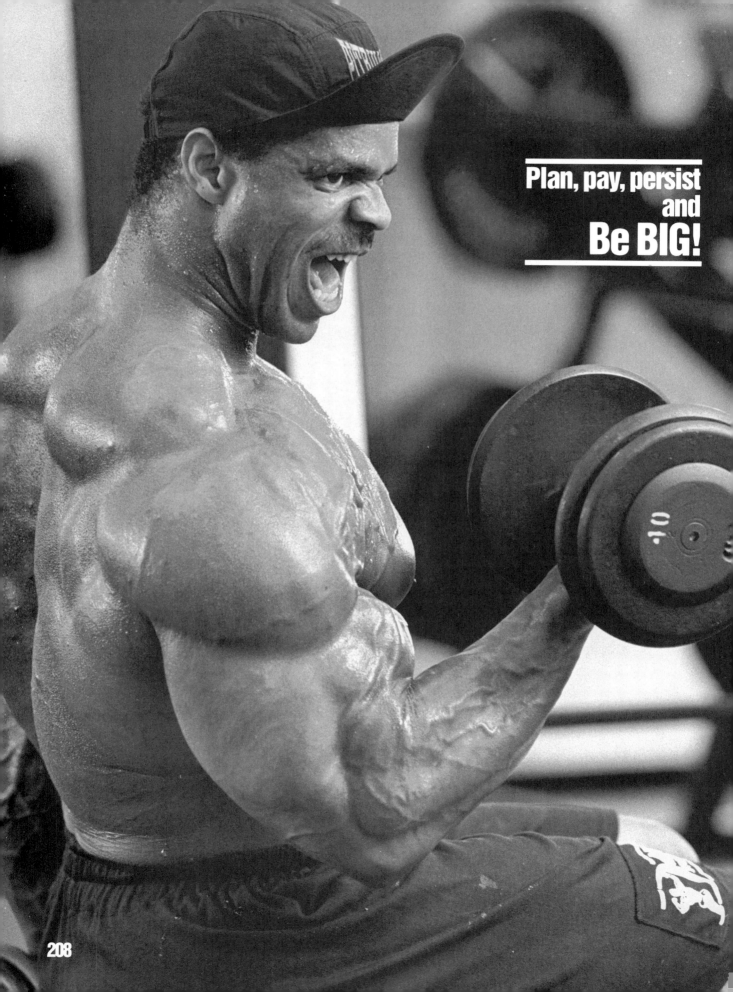

Plan, pay, persist and **Be BIG!**